# The MYSTERY

## of sustained
## weight loss
## And you thought it
## was
## impossible!?

Dr Stephen K Fairley

# Chapters

So despite this study, and literally hundreds like it, we still continue to suggest dieting is a good idea?!

If you want to succeed in sustained weight loss you need to make a *lifestyle change,* from the moment you get up in the morning to the time you go to bed in the evening. You change your eating habits as well as many other things and you do so for good. You need to make these changes for the rest of your life.

You need to take a look at what you are doing and turn over a new leaf. Everything from how you perceive yourself, what you put in your mouth, what is actually available to eat in your place of residence, your exercise plans, your daily habits, what you do in your work and leisure time needs review. This is only the beginning of the list. You need to change the way you think and feel about weight loss and your whole outlook on the issue needs to be addressed.

This begins with education about what you should be eating and what you should not – in other words, understanding what the building blocks of the food you are putting in your mouth are made of, running through to how you perceive yourself. The aim of this book is to educate you about the very real problem at hand and to take you through a step-wise, easy to follow approach for confronting and addressing this problem in the long term.

In short, you are starting a new chapter in the book on the rest of your life, and a longer happier more fulfilling life it is likely to be. This is not for the faint hearted. It is not going to be easy and you are going to have to be committed. However, the good news is, in the long term it is going to come naturally. Your obesity and all that goes with it will be a thing of the past.

# CHAPTER 1

## Obesity in our society

IF WE ARE to discuss obesity and weight loss we need some definitions to ensure we are all talking about the same thing. The simplest method for doing this, which I suspect you are all familiar with, is the BMI or body mass index. This is a simple mathematical calculation of your weight in kg divided by your height in metres squared. Any type of measurement we use here will have some problems and the issue with BMI is that it does not take into account different body builds. Someone who literally does have "bigger bones", as opposed to the numerous people out there who simply think they do, will have a higher BMI and not necessarily be overweight. In addition, if one goes to the gym a lot and develops a large muscle mass, you may similarly have a high BMI without actually being overweight in terms of relative fat mass.

Putting these issues aside, it is a reasonable measure when applied across the board to a population.

Now a "normal" or "healthy" BMI for an adult is said to lie in the range of 18-25.

If your BMI is between 25 and 30 we use the term "overweight".

If your BMI is greater than 30 we use the term "obese", and so it goes on with other less complimentary terms used for higher numbers. Remember however this does not take into account different races and builds. Someone of European background with 25% of their body weight as fat has a BMI of about 30. Someone of Chinese background with 25% body fat has a BMI of 23-24, when clearly they have the same degree of obesity as the European. For this reason your percentage body fat would be a better measure, but it is harder to estimate, so generally we will work with BMI. What is your value?

If you do not know your height, it is in your wallet on your driver's license, and the scales are in the bathroom! Your smart phone has a calculator on it in case you pretend not to have noticed this.

Waist to hip circumference is a simpler, and probably better, way of assessing if you are overweight in all the wrong places. This has significant health implications as discussed in the next chapter. Take a tape measure and put it around your abdomen. Measure your waist, which is just above your umbilicus (belly button), and put this measurement over the measurement taken from around your hips. The hip measurement includes your buttocks at the level of the maximum size. Keep the tape parallel with the floor. If the ratio is greater than 0.9 in males or 0.85 in females you are in trouble.

How do you take the measurements when your umbilicus is hanging below the level of your hips? Clearly the issue is academic. You don't need to bother with any measurement at all.

Now when discussing the issue of obesity at the level of a society or particular population, the people most published about seem to be those in the USA. Admittedly obesity is a very real issue there. However, in Australia, where I am based, we are just as bad, if not worse, in some subsets of the population.

The data for the USA comes from national surveys of height and weight of the population, or more particularly the "National Health and Nutrition Examination Survey" or "NHANES". These surveys suggest that things started to change in the late 1970s or early 1980s with figures increasing by as much as 1% per year until early this century. Now 1% per year may not sound like much, but it means that over that period the vast majority of the US population were shifted from normal weight into the overweight or above category. Hence, no matter how you would like to put it politely, now nearly all of them are "fat". The same is true of Australia and many other countries.

The NHANES data for 2009-2010 show that for adult (older than 20) males, 69.2% are overweight or obese, and for females it is 64.5% of the population. To make matters worse, there is a rising trend with age. The older people are, the higher is their BMI. If you look at those over 60 years of age the figures are 76.5% for males and 73.5% for females. In other words, only one in four of this age group are in the healthy weight range. As their muscles weaken with age they are even less likely to be able to look after themselves than normal weight older people, placing further stress on societies' resources. The BMI of children is also rising and we know that large children make large adults.

There is one positive point in assessing the data from the 1960s to today, and that is that the rate at which we are all getting fatter seems to be slowing, at least in so called developed countries. In the last 10 years only men seemed to be getting fatter, with less change in the women. This may in part be due to our obsession, in Western culture, with trying, usually unsuccessfully, to look thin and fit rather than fat. There is generally a negative social stigma attached to obesity in these cultures. Obese people tend to be viewed as lazy and stupid, however unfair, incorrect and insulting this may be.

_Katherine M. Flegal, PhD et al., JAMA, February 1, 2012—Vol. 307, No. 5._

The reduction in the rate of weight gain does not apply to the developing world, with much of the developing world in hot pursuit, staging their own obesity epidemics and following trends set in the developed world. Just 30 years ago the World Health Organisation's primary agendas in poorer countries were feeding children and fighting infection. We still have starving children in many countries and unfortunately we are not winning on the infection control front either, with HIV infection and multidrug resistant malaria and TB taking a firmer hold.

There is concern now however for another serious health problem overwhelming the health care resources in these countries, with the obesity pandemic sweeping the world. It began in the USA, swept across Europe and is now involving the second and third world countries, including some very poor countries in Africa, albeit mainly in the urban populations here. There is another problem when considering the peoples who have come from more "primitive", for want of a better word, societies, and where this epidemic is leading them. The genes which code for increased likelihood of survival in a period of famine are, as one might expect, more common in these people. To look at this another way, all those who did not have these genes died off in famines in the past and only those with what we describe as the "thrifty phenotype" remain. If they were motor vehicles, everyone would want to buy them because they use less fuel. Unfortunately however, in a time of plenty these genes make them more sensitive to the negative effects of weight gain, with dire consequences, as I will discuss later. I am talking about groups like Australian Aborigines, New Zealand Maoris, North American Indians, Black Africans, Asians ... in short, most of the world's population. So you see we do have a problem.

The obvious question here is why is this happening to us all? Why me? There are a number of theories. However, one just has to look at the equation of what's going in and what's coming out in terms of energy balance and it is relatively easy to understand at least part of the problem. There has been a dramatic reduction in the price and availability of highly refined oils and carbohydrates from fast food outlets and supermarkets in the past 30 years. Aggressive marketing of fast, high calorie foods at a cheap price with easy availability leads to one thing: increased consumption. So what have we done to balance the increased intake of calories? If the answer was nothing this would be bad enough, but it is worse than nothing! At the same time we have actually reduced our energy expenditure. All of a sudden (in evolutionary terms) we have motorised personal transport, usually a car, so we no longer have to walk or ride a bike to work or to the bus or railway station, we just walk out our front door and hop in a car. Then when we get to work it gets worse again. Instead of working in field growing corn or digging holes we sit, usually in front of a computer screen, for hours on end.

That's okay: once we get home we will do some exercise, won't we? Well, one would hope so, but once home and tired from sitting and concentrating all day we are then seduced by the TV, computer games or the internet. A bit tired tonight to cook a healthy meal and have to go out later, so thank goodness for the pizza store on the corner to get something convenient to eat! Come to think of it, I had pizza last night: I'd better have the fried chicken and chips from the store on the opposite corner tonight. A balanced diet is so important!

Luckily however our bodies have an in-built setting for our "ideal weight" and they actively try to resist significant weight gain by increasing your metabolic rate to burn off more calories and secreting hormones to reduce your appetite, among other things. Hopefully that will work to stop us getting fat, and it does to a point. The problem is, however, that if you try hard enough you overwhelm your defences. Slowly but surely they give in. You may only gain 1-2 kg per year, but when you multiply this out over 20 years you are putting on some serious weight. The problem then is that our body resets its ideal weight at the new level. When you then try to lose weight it uses the same mechanisms that resisted your weight gain, only in reverse, to drag you back up again, very effectively reducing your weight loss. This is why it is so hard to lose the weight!

Our body image also plays a role in our response to being overweight. If we or our family and friends don't see there is a problem, why try to fix it?

Some cultures view obesity as a positive thing, associated with power, beauty and wealth, and one only has to look to some of the island nations in the Pacific Ocean to see what happens if you combine this belief with the other issues already mentioned. In the pacific nation of Nauru, even 20 years ago in 1994, 80% of the adult population were in the obese range with a BMI of 30 or greater. I dare not try to find any more recent statistics on this society.

---

*Andrew M Prentice, International Journal of Epidemiology 2006; 35: 93–99.*

In terms of the question of history and "why are we all so fat?" there are clearly many issues, but there is one thing that stands out and may be very relevant. In 1977 the USA imposed a tariff on imported sugar, significantly increasing the cost of sucrose or table sugar to twice that of the global price. The sugar was used to sweeten foods and the processed food makers went looking for an alternative. Unfortunately for us they found one: high fructose corn syrup. To make matters worse, the USA government paid subsidies to corn growers to keep the cost of corn low at the same time as the food industry, with the help of the Japanese, worked out how to convert surplus waste corn into a sweet syrup on a massive scale. As always, large amounts of money were to be made by all involved in the process to keep the ball rolling. Consequently high fructose syrup replaced cane sugar in processed food. Not only was it much cheaper than sucrose or table sugar, it was sweeter too, a double bonus. It very rapidly found its way into soft drinks, confectionaries, breakfast cereals, bread, lunch meats, yogurt, fast foods including the hamburger bun and patty, and almost anything else sweet you care to mention. The problem with the sugar fructose is, as I will explain later in the book, there is no off switch for your eating when you consume it. If anything, it keeps encouraging you to come back for more and does not switch off or supress your appetite. It is also preferentially turned into fat in all the wrong places, such as your liver and your abdomen, with potentially bad consequences for your general health. Heard of diseases like diabetes before?

So when did the obesity epidemic begin? The answer is about 1980. When did high fructose corn syrup (HFCS) begin being placed in huge amounts in the food you are eating? The answer is about 1980. Is there any correlation between the amount of

HFCS consumed in a society and the levels of obesity? Yes, a straight line graph: if you double one you double the other. In other words, societies that consume twice as much corn syrup have twice as much obesity in their society. Draw your own conclusions. Do not be fooled by the misinformation coming out of the multibillion dollar HFCS suppliers and food processors to tell you this is just a coincidence. The sounds they are making are almost identical to the tobacco industry, who for at least 20 years after tobacco was proven to cause cancer, continued to deny it and try to falsify all claims by medical science to the contrary. Why would they do that? I'm sure it has nothing to do with money! If you go back and look at the way the tobacco industry behaved after the association between lung cancer and smoking was proven, the food industry is doing the same thing with respect to processed foods and the obesity epidemic. They say it is all because of lack of exercise and nothing to do with their healthy naturally sweetened foods, and they hope you believe them and keep buying. Well, that has been proven to be far from accurate. If there is a problem, it is your fault not theirs and it is your right to buy anything you like, so please buy some more ....

Something else happened at about 1980, around the time of the onset of the obesity epidemic, and it too was about company profits and not about your health. The makers of fast foods realised a few things about the human psyche. Firstly, they realised people did not want to look greedy going back for a second serving of chips or another hamburger or soft drink, so they trialled increasing serving sizes that allowed them to charge more and maximise their profits. The second issue related to the relative pricing of the increased serve. They would offer you twice as many chips but for only 50% more in price, so it appeared you were getting twice as much for only one and a half times as much cost to you, which of course you were! This was the beginning of the concept of supersizing, which took off in the USA and rapidly spread to the rest of the world. Customers swallowed the bait hook, line and sinker! And why wouldn't they? They were getting much better value for money, and the fast food outlets pushed this concept for all it was worth. Now what the customer did not realise is that the cost of the increased size portion is almost nothing to the fast food seller. Their primary costs are the cost of the labour serving you the chips, the cost of electricity or gas running the deep fryer and hot plates and the cost of leasing the building you are standing in – not to mention the cost of advertising to make sure you do not miss out on this wonderful deal! Putting a few extra slices of potato in the bag is only about a 5% increase in cost to them, leaving them with a sudden 45% increase in profit while you think it is you who are getting the benefit! All the other costs to them stayed the same! Think about it.

Now when it comes to the soft drink or soda, things get even better for the people selling them to the gullible public. They give you twice the serve for only 50% more cost, but it costs them only about another 1% or less and the other 49% extra money you just gave them goes in the equation as pure profit to the company selling you the soft drink. Is that really great value for you? I have already explained that the corn syrup used to sweeten the soft drink costs almost nothing, and how much do you think the extra water and colouring costs? This has been milked for all it is worth at outrageous profits to the fast food makers and food manufacturers in general. The size of a soft drink began at about 300 mls in the 1970s and in some fast food stores you can now get sizes up to about 2 litres. Now 2 litres of soft drink contains about 50, yes that's right, FIFTY teaspoons of sugar, in one drink! Now where do you think that sugar goes after you swallow it? That's right, straight to your abdomen where it is turned into fat.

Now I'm sure that you think logically that if you have more food now at less cost you will be better off because you don't have to eat again for longer and you will eat less at your next meal. Wrong again, and on both counts! If you eat a larger serve of this high sugar, high salt and high fat meal for lunch, the evidence is that it has no effect on the size of evening meal you consume; this remains unchanged. All that has changed is that you got far more calories that day.

The food processing industry, again with its billions of dollars in financial reserves, tried very hard to counter the negative press on this issue that was glaringly apparent to a number of health professionals. Early attempts to publish negatively on this issue were just swept under the carpet. After all, these companies were giving large amounts of money to politicians, so they had a right to get something for their money, didn't they? I mean that's only fair, isn't it? I would use the term "corrupt", but again, you make up your own mind. With the public catching on, at last they came up with another idea for giving the customer "extra value for money", just what the customer was wanting. This time they called them "value meals". Sound familiar? Now you could get your burger, extra-large fries and extra-large drink for much less than the cost of adding up each one individually as you had to in the past. You may even get a free soft serve ice cream. What fantastic value for your money! You would have to be an idiot to buy them individually, wouldn't you? Well, it appeared that way as the "value meals" came to make up about half of the profits from these fast food outlets, adding further vast quantities of profits for the companies involved. The only problem was for the person who had just bought the "extra value meal". They felt they could not waste this food and drink so they consumed it all, when they may not have bought all of it if it was only sold in individual items. The fast food companies didn't care – remember, it cost them almost nothing to give you the extra parts of the meal – and their profits were soaring! Now if you feel I am overdoing this in terms of questioning the morality of the companies involved then I think you are sadly mistaken. Perhaps we should be discuss the morals of these companies directly targeting children in the advertising, or putting toys for the children in their "happy meals", to encourage the children to pressure their parents to buy these products. As I am sure you are aware, this obesity epidemic involves not only adults but children also. It looks like the health effects of being obese from childhood are dire and fat children almost invariably make fat adults. Again the food processors have tried to mislead the public, saying it is all the parents' fault, or it is all about the children doing less exercise, but don't be fooled, at least with the latter fact. Children in studies are doing about the same amount of exercise overall as they did in the past; it is the dramatic increase in calories they are taking in causing the obesity, not the lack of exercise. There is some evidence however that once they are grossly overweight they have more trouble being able to exercise. In other words, the obesity causes the lack of exercise rather than the lack of exercise causing obesity, as you are all led to believe. Things are not always what they seem. Advertising targeting children continues, because it works and it increases profits.

Now if you think you are safe if you stay away from fast food outlets then I'm afraid you need to think again. The fast food outlets help you save time, which I'm sure you all agree is a scarce commodity in our busy lifestyle. The supermarkets you all shop in are there to help too! They save you time as well because they sell you processed foods, which makes a busy lifestyle much easier, doesn't it? All you have to do is put it in the microwave and peel off the plastic once it is cooked or just add milk or water. The trouble with processed food, generally speaking, is that it is loaded with hidden calories, some of them very very unhealthy, such as trans-fatty acids and fructose. You don't even know what these substances are, do you? Surely this does not apply to my toasted muesli and low fat yogurt, does it? This is why it is so important you read the rest of this book. Supermarkets are good at one thing: supersizing you. You were much better off when the markets were fresh food markets. Remember these? Your grandparents and great grandparents used to shop at them. Do they look obese in their old photos?

At the risk of boring you, I am going to give you one message over and over again in this book. Don't let other people "process" your food for you, do it yourself! Learn to interpret this word truthfully. When they say "processed" they actually mean "poisoned". Don't believe me? Look at the people standing around you.

Do not be fooled into thinking big brother or your government will take care of you in this world where there is a quick buck to be made selling you or your family this type of food. Surely they wouldn't put my family's health before money, would they? What do you think? It is up to you to look after yourself and your family in this "brave new world" where money rules. You may not have to worry about the lions and tigers any more, but there are still very dangerous threats to you and your family's wellbeing out there. Learn to recognise them.

We were designed by nature or evolution to live in a cave, run around hunting, climb trees, and search for berries and other foods in the jungle for a living. In evolutionary terms however the change from then to now occurred in the blink of an eye and neither our bodies nor our genes have had time to adapt to the change, with the obvious result hanging over your belt buckle. Our bodies are not designed to live in modern society and if we want to remain healthy in this environment that is "foreign" or "alien" to our genetic makeup we have to think about what we are doing where eating and exercising is concerned.

So if we think we understand part of the "why" we are getting obese as a society, the next question is the where of "where are we going?" Well, I do not believe anyone can see into the future. However, health consequences of the obesity epidemic are almost beyond belief and I will explain why in another chapter. This is very serious stuff and on its current trajectory will completely overwhelm the health care resources in developed and developing countries in the very near future. This is NOT sustainable. We MUST find a way to turn back and we are rapidly running out of time.

# CHAPTER 2

# The consequences of obesity

*So what is all the hype about? What does it matter if I am considered over-weight? I know I am not fat: just look at all my friends, they are all much bigger than I am.*

WELL I AM glad you are comfortable in your own skin and don't think there is an issue. At least you are able to feel relaxed about the issue at hand. What issue was that anyway?

That is how we are all encouraged to think in our society, isn't it? After all, it is just not right if someone is seen to criticise you is it? You might have to go looking for a lawyer to sue them for bullying or slander, even if they, possibly being your doctor, were simply trying to help you. Nice to know we are all being politically, socially and emotionally correct and aware, isn't it?

Well I am sorry to say you have come to the wrong doctor. I tell my patients the truth and do not tiptoe around offering a whole lot of vague waffly niceties while trying to make them feel good about themselves. You have probably already picked this up!

When they leave they hopefully understand the issue being discussed and what needs to be done about it, regardless of whether their mood is higher or lower and regardless of whether they are likely to act on the advice or education they have received. Unfortunately, you cannot get through to everyone. Some of them don't come back to see me again. They go and see nice doctors.

I see my primary role as that of providing EDUCATION and MOTIVATION. After 30 years of talking to patients in consultation and surveying the results of my discussions I believe a direct approach is the best one. Sure, it does not work for everyone: some people already know everything, so what could they possibly learn from their doctor? Some patients need a different approach to increase the likelihood of getting the message across. I would like to make the point that I never try to offend people for the sake of it, only in the context of trying to motivate them when all else fails. Anger is a very powerful tool to motivate people. I am very happy for the result of a discussion with a patient to be, "I'll show him!"

So if being overweight is not an issue for you, then might I respectfully suggest it will help if you are religious and believe that when you die you are going to a better place. You will be boarding that train a lot earlier than you may have realised. If you are obese not only do you get preferential treatment to board the early train, you get to board the slow and painful train too, lucky you! Unlike the express train, your train not only has bad suspension to jar your arthritis, it will make many stops at other stations on the way to pick up high blood pressure, high cholesterol, diabetes, heart disease, strokes and many cancers on its way to the terminal station where you get off.

I would love to have a faith and feel jealous of those of you who are lucky enough to do so, as losing loved ones for a start would be a lot easier, knowing they were going to be in a better place. As for me, however, with no idea where I am going to be going, I would like to stay here in the present for as long as possible. I am in no hurry to leave on the early train, and most of my patients are not either when the options are put to them. The issue is simply how to motivate them to ensure they don't buy the wrong tickets at the station!

There are exceptions to every rule, but just think about how many fat 90 year olds you have met. Don't want to live to 90, you say? Well I am talking just as much about the quality of your life as the quantity in this discussion.

The consequences of obesity are best summarised in the term "The Metabolic Syndrome". It is not perfect but is probably the best model to describe this. The definition is three of the five following conditions: obesity around the middle of the body or trunk, high blood pressure, raised blood sugar, raised triglycerides or blood fats, and low high density lipoprotein or good cholesterol. This could also be called "Medical conditions associated with obesity". It is essentially a syndrome of "carbohydrate poisoning" or if you like an "exercise deficiency state", depending on which side of the equation you look at. Too much carbohydrate goes in on the left side of the equation and too little exercise comes out on the right side. What is the thing sitting right in the middle of this equation getting bigger and bigger because this equation is not balanced? No prizes for guessing this, it is obviously YOU. This syndrome is best thought of as a combination of these two issues. It can usually be cured by tackling either side of the equation but most effectively by tackling both sides.

When one sits and tries to honestly list the diseases associated with the metabolic syndrome one quickly realises they are so numerous that perhaps it would be easier to list those diseases not yet known to be associated! The syndrome and its consequences account for a very large component of the health care budgets in the Western world. The syndrome is the reason many are predicting that we or our children may be the first generation in hundreds of years to have a shorter life expectancy than their parents. Many thousands or tens of thousands of people across the globe die prematurely every day from the consequences of this disease, but does anyone seem to care? What if 1000 people died in a plane or train crash, then all of a sudden it is across all media interfaces. No, this is the silent killer lurking there waiting for you. No one talks about it and it hardly gets mentioned in the media at all. It most certainly does not get the airplay it deserves. If it did I would not be writing this book. The ignorant and uninformed call it "natural causes". The educated, hopefully including you, know there is no such thing as "natural causes". Everybody dies from something. It is much easier however to use a term like "natural causes" when your 60-year-old partner or parent dies unexpectedly from a heart attack, a stroke or bowel cancer, than admitting his or her death could possibly have been prevented and they may have had another 10, 20 or 30 happy productive years. This is serious stuff so please wake up and think about what is being said here.

You do not need to have a PhD in maths to understand this equation. At least 50% of people with obesity develop features of the metabolic syndrome; the bigger you are the greater the risk. Many of the features of the metabolic syndrome become more common as part of natural aging, obesity just allows you to bring them on 10, 20 or 30 years earlier than was otherwise going to be the case.

There is no question your genes play an important part here in predisposing you to many of the conditions associated with the metabolic syndrome. *Predisposition* and *Causation* are different things and if we are to succeed here you must stop confusing them. You did not get your type 2 diabetes from your father. You got the predisposition to developing it if you chose to do so.

This is a very important concept and I am going to go over it multiple times. If you already have a firm grasp on the genetic issues here that's great. If you don't then stay with me as I walk you through it. It is critically important you understand this concept as if you do not you will think you are powerless. You will not make the necessary changes to improve your situation. The game will be over before it has even begun.

The metabolic syndrome, or many of its components are not forced on you by your genes in the majority of cases. You have to actively choose to accept them yourself, they are not your parents fault. It is a bit like choosing extras with a meal, you could have a side salad or chips with your meal, just like you can choose to add type two diabetes and high blood pressure to your current list of medical problems. Your choice not fate. You are the one in control.

Your genes are associated with your risk or likelihood for developing these diseases and your genes are complex and multiple, but this concept is not.

Let us look at something which is conveyed by your genes such as the colour of your skin as one example. The metabolic syndrome and all of its components are like sunburn in this example.

If you are born with fair or white skin as opposed to dark skin, this is likely genetic and related to your parents, no argument. Just because you have fair skin does not mean you have to get sunburnt! To achieve this you must obviously go out in the sun, your choice! Sure you are more likely to get sunburnt if you go in the sun than the person with the dark skin in this example, however they can get sunburnt too, they just have to try harder. The *predisposition* to getting sunburnt is genetic, the *cause* of the sunburn is definitely not. The latter is related to your behaviour, not to your genes or your parents. In other words I say again, you are the one in control. Your father or mother did not cause you to get sunburnt, you did! You went outside in the sun! Your choice!

In a similar fashion, the predisposition to getting the components of the metabolic syndrome such as diabetes is genetically determined. Actually choosing to accept it is not. It may be difficult when you live in a society where food is plentiful and your lifestyle makes exercise difficult, or if you live where the sun shines intensely as in the previous example. It is far from impossible to avoid the sunburn or the diabetes. The fact that you are born with a predisposition to diabetes does not mean you have it. To collect the diabetes you must either overeat and/or fail to exercise. To collect the sunburn you must go out in the sun. Neither will happen without input from you. You are to blame and you are the only one who can reverse the situation. So please get out of the sun!

You can think of this as being a bit like a seesaw where food is put on one end and exercise on the other. If you balance the two ends it stays horizontal and you stay well. If the end with the food on it touches the ground you lose and you develop diabetes, your choice. To stop this happening you can take the food off one end (eat less, particularly carbohydrate) or you can put more exercise on the other end. No one else as can do this for you, you must take charge and do it yourself. Don't be passive and just blame your parents, they didn't have any say in their genes either. You must understand this to be proactive. You must be a player here, you are not a spectator. Get off the couch, turn off the TV and go for a walk.

The syndrome begins with slow gradual weight gain that causes a condition called insulin resistance. Insulin resistance means your body is resistant to the effects of insulin so you need a higher level of insulin to achieve the same result in terms of a normal blood sugar. Insulin is the primary hormone or messenger in the blood that controls the level of blood sugar. You would not be aware of anything at this stage. However, it may be notable that you are beginning to develop an increase in your girth and if you had an ultrasound of the liver the report would read "increased echogenicity in keeping with early fatty infiltration". There is nothing magical about fatty liver disease, it is just a marker of abdominal obesity. If you put on weight around the middle you put it on in your liver and you are likely to develop insulin resistance. The rest follows as you slip on the slope of the mountain and descend rapidly in an avalanche towards the valley floor below.

When discussing fat in the body it is important to understand that we generally describe two types of obesity or excessive fat distribution. The fat around the middle or abdomen is the more dangerous fat in terms of the risk of the metabolic syndrome and premature death. This is the fat on the inside or the *visceral fat.* This fat is very metabolically active and has numerous effects on the rest of the body. It is the first fat to go if you exercise or diet as it is the first fat called on to supply the body with energy in a time of need, when you run out of glucose or sugar in your liver. The second type of fat is under the skin, so called *subcutaneous fat* or fat on the outside. This type of fat is around your bottom, legs, breasts, arms and neck and is much harder to lose. Sure, you will burn it off eventually if you don't eat, but it has to be a long time since the last rain for this to occur. Those of you who have tried seriously dieting know this.

An example of people who are *predisposed* to the metabolic syndrome or if you like are at very high risk, people from southern Asia fit this profile and have a so called *thrifty phenotype.* They tend to put fat on in the abdomen without necessarily having to be very overweight in terms of BMI. As a result they develop the metabolic syndrome at a lower weight. Remember this is similar to the example of people with fair skin getting sunburnt more easily than those with dark skin. If you wonder if you are in this category, if your parents or siblings develop diabetes without being very overweight it is likely you too carry this genetic *thrifty phenotype* and are at increased risk of these associated diseases. It is too late to do anything about your parents by the time you read this, so there is no point trying. In the future, however, we might be able to change our genes. The other thing strongly associated with increasing risk of the metabolic syndrome is age. As we can as yet do nothing about this, I will stick to worrying about things we can change: your weight, your diet and your participation in exercise.

Without worrying about strict medical definitions, the metabolic syndrome is a combination of fat in the abdomen and resistance to the effect of insulin. As mentioned, fatty liver is one of the earliest markers. The metabolically active fat in the abdomen produces many things, including inflammatory cytokines or messengers, so called adipokines as they come from adipose (fat) tissue. These cause inflammation throughout the body as well as contributing to the insulin resistance discussed above. Inflammation is not a good thing (just think about how you feel with the flu) as it damages other cells. One of the cell types of concern here is the endothelium or "Teflon like" lining cells on the inside of arteries, which are there to stop blood sticking to the walls. If the blood products stick, you either get gradual thickening of the walls of the arteries over the long term causing gradual blockage. If you get a blood clot and sudden blockage the result depends on where the artery is. If it is in your head some of your brain dies, a so called cerebrovascular accident or "stroke"; if it is in your heart it is a heart attack. If it is your leg, they often have to cut this off below the blockage. This is an amputation associated with what we call peripheral vascular disease.

Inflammation associated with your fat abdomen probably contributes to other things you haven't even thought about. One that you probably don't know about is osteoarthritis. You thought your joints just wore out from all the exercise you did, didn't you? If you are more honest, perhaps you felt they wore out because they were not designed to carry the weight of two people around. Well, you are partly wrong on both counts, so you don't need to feel proud or guilty! The correlation between exercise without joint injury and loss of the joint cartilage, which keeps it lubricated and moving, is poor. The correlation between the metabolic syndrome and the loss of joint cartilage and subsequent joint destruction is strong. In fact, if you plot the number of components of the metabolic syndrome someone has against the severity of their osteoarthritis or joint destruction on a graph, it is a straight line. The worse the metabolic syndrome, the worse the joint disease. Far fewer thin people, who have not had joint injuries, end up having to have their knee and hip joints replaced. This is assuming they do not have the metabolic syndrome. If you have ever had a joint replaced you will know what a huge undertaking it is, especially if something goes wrong like infection and the new joint has to be removed.

You can look at this another way and compare disease of the lining of the carotid artery (running to your brain) with severity of osteoarthritis in the hands as an alternative example. The disease in the carotid artery is a marker for severity in the metabolic syndrome. Again, there seems to be a strong association: the worse the osteoarthritis in the hands, the worse the artery disease in the neck. You don't walk on your hands, and this arthritis does not correlate with you having been a hard manual worker. The osteoarthritis seems to be an inflammatory condition associated with the increased inflammation in the body, the inflammation being associated with the metabolic syndrome. The essential cartilage in the joint just dissolves away in the inflammation, a bit like dissolving something in strong acid. When it's gone, it's gone, and the joint surgery is the only option to get reasonable function back. The new joint will never be anything like as good as the original joint. Now the metabolic syndrome may not be the whole story when it comes to osteoarthritis but it is clearly contributing factor over which you have some control. You cannot undo old joint injuries or change your genes or your age so I suggest we focus on things we can do something about.

Hopefully if we start early your need for joint replacements may be reduced in the future.

_Hashimora, J Rheum 2011. Jonsson ARD 2012._

These inflammatory mediators may also be involved in premature dementia and more rapid ageing as well many other things we are only just learning about.

With increasing weight and increasing insulin resistance your insulin levels rise to Olympic proportions in an attempt to keep your blood sugar in the normal range. Your pancreas is responsible for producing insulin, and this situation is a bit like indefinitely whipping a horse galloping along the track until finally it collapses and falls over. At this time the pancreas says, "Okay, I give up, I can't do this anymore!" Congratulations, you've got diabetes! This is type 2 diabetes, usually accomplished after years of concerted effort on behalf of the patient, where the insulin levels are high, at least initially. It is not to be confused with type 1 diabetes which occurs out of the blue in young people, through no fault of their own and possibly triggered by an infection.

So you still feel it is unreasonable for me to blame you for your type 2 diabetes?

Did I hear you say it's genetic, your genes did it not you? That's odd, I didn't know genes could overeat, fail to exercise or sunbake, but I suppose you learn something new every day. Well, I'm sorry for dwelling on this, but you are not listening and I say again, in the vast majority of cases of type 2 diabetes it is your fault and it could have been avoided. This might seem a bit harsh in a day and age where it seems at times (to the doctors) as if patients think nothing is ever their fault and they come in demanding a quick fix. Type 2 diabetes can, as I've said, probably be cured if you act early. It is up to you to fix it. Your doctor is only there to try and help, as is the advice in this book. If you will not take ownership for these issues, be they sunburn or diabetes, then how are we to go about fixing them? Don't forget to pick up your early train ticket if you are not interested in making any effort here.

The other common medical conditions that we said were part of the metabolic syndrome were raised cholesterol, raised triglycerides or fats in the blood and high blood pressure. Sure, I agree your parents, by sharing their genes with you, may have put you at increased risk of developing these conditions also. "I got high blood pressure or high cholesterol from my parents!" Sound familiar? Like diabetes, this does not always mean you are powerless to do anything about it, so stop looking for excuses! Look to yourself first, not your doctor to fix this, but please do see your doctor and discuss this issue with them, they will encourage you. Many of the end results here are one-way streets and we don't want you turning into them unnecessarily.

All of these conditions are associated with an increased risk of vascular (arterial) disease, particularly heart attacks, strokes and peripheral vascular disease, and treatment reduces this risk. Sadly in medicine, instead of treating the cause of the whole condition, we treat all the side issues and end results. In other words, instead of encouraging exercise and weight loss we give you 1-3 tablets for your blood pressure, 1-3 tablets for your diabetes, another for your cholesterol, some aspirin to make the blood less sticky, another tablet to treat your arthritis ...

How many tablets was that? How many are you taking? The reason we as doctors do this is not because we want you to keep coming back for medication. It is because we know after years of trying to get you to exercise and lose weight, we almost invariably fail. It is like banging one's head against a brick wall. Eventually the headache is so bad you just give up. The doctors are human, after all. I am hoping this book will be more effective if you understand the issues involved and where you are headed. Then you can deal with these diseases and hopefully cure some or all of them. Until then keep taking your tablets as they do reduce your risk, and never stop them without discussing the issue with your doctor.

Now I want to come back to fatty liver disease or fatty liver in more detail, having skipped over this initially. It is one of the first things we find in this condition but is by no means the least. Roughly half of the population have this condition and the incidence is rising at an alarming rate, with all the associated diseases already described. The medical term for this is non-alcoholic fatty liver disease, as under the microscope it looks identical to fatty liver disease related to alcohol, which is another topic altogether. The disease is much more of a worry if there is associated inflammation, and the larger you are the more likely it is that there is going to be associated inflammation present on blood testing or on looking under the microscope at a piece of your liver. Ouch! Did you just stick a needle in my liver to take a biopsy? If you have the more severe form of this disease there is about a 50% chance you are going to die from cirrhosis of the liver, with or without this being complicated by liver cancer. You can easily achieve this without a drop of alcohol ever touching your lips. Advanced age, diabetes, a BMI of >28 and a large amount of abdominal fat all increase your risk substantially. You can't change your age, but you can change all the other factors here.

Now for those of you who miss out on dying from liver failure or liver cancer, both of which are strongly associated with the metabolic syndrome, all is not lost as there is still a good chance you will die from cardiovascular diseases such as a stroke or heart attack or from many other cancers. This may occur while you are having dialysis because of your kidney failure. Sorry, did I forget to mention you are also at risk of kidney failure? This is okay though as you have three options here: death, dialysis every 3 days, or a kidney transplant if you are lucky enough to find someone to give you another kidney.

So what is the commonest cause of chronic kidney failure requiring dialysis or renal transplantation in our society? Could it be type 2 diabetes? What was the cause of type 2 diabetes? Wasn't it the metabolic syndrome? Yes it was and those at the most risk of the metabolic syndrome, especially some subgroups mentioned such as Australian Aboriginals are the at the greatest risk of developing renal failure associated with their diabetes.

So I would pose the question: does it make financial or humanitarian sense to step in at the end of someone's life with a dialysis machine as a band aid for a disease that is by that time incurable? Should we not be directing our health care dollars towards preventing these diseases in the first place? This syndrome is particularly unfair as it is targeting the most vulnerable and uninformed groups in our society.

Remember, this was mostly preventable in two ways: diet and exercise.

As if things are not bad enough already, I am not finished. I have alluded to the fact that there are many cancers associated with obesity and the metabolic syndrome. These are related to many parts of your body and you would be surprised that the relative risk of developing conditions such as breast cancer are made much higher simply by being overweight. Breast cancer, like all cancers, is a terrible thing. In non-smoking women it is the commonest cause of cancer related death. The risk of developing breast cancer is as high as 1 in 8 in the United States.

The data on how many lives screening with x-ray (mammography) for breast cancer saves suggests that at best it may reduce the risk of death by 25%. Other studies are less complimentary about this form of screening, with concerns that the x-rays may increase your risk of cancer. As there is as much as a 50% increased risk of breast cancer in obese post-menopausal women, don't we have other options that are possibly more effective?

What was that about prevention being better than cure? This does not apply to all cases of breast cancer, I am simply making the statistical observation that if we could cure obesity we may have a much larger reduction in breast cancer deaths than we do through screening with mammography.

Now if we go on to consider the commonest cause of cancer related death among men who don't smoke, bowel cancer holds this prize. Around 25%-50% of these cases of bowel cancer are potentially associated with the obesity epidemic, with obesity being the single largest recognisable risk factor. The trouble with these figures is that cancers take 20 years or so to develop, and we do not know what the future holds as the obesity epidemic is a very recent thing. It could get much worse in the near future!

Other relatively common cancers with an increased incidence in obesity include a rough doubling of the risk of cancer of the uterus, gall bladder and lower oesophagus. Cancers of the stomach (upper), pancreas, prostate and kidney are all increased. This is far from a complete list, I am only discussing relatively common cancers here.

Other non-malignant but very important diseases strongly associated with obesity and the metabolic syndrome are sleep apnoea syndrome, polycystic ovarian syndrome and gout. These are huge problems for society as a whole, in terms of resultant days lost from productive work and fatal motor car accidents, not to mention the personal suffering of those with the conditions.

So you don't have to worry about being fat at all, do you? As long as you are happy in your own skin there is nothing else to worry about – or is there?

Is it not time to consider tackling these issues at the level of society with prevention where possible, rather than a doctor trying to pick up the pieces at the end? Until that time comes, I am hoping I can motivate you and give advice to help you achieve permanent weight loss.

Now once you are overweight, have diabetes, high blood pressure, and high cholesterol, and see your doctor about these issues, you will no doubt have been put on multiple medications for your problems to "control" these diseases you have developed with ageing and weight gain. The reason we use these medications is because all of the diseases associated with the metabolic syndrome increase your mortality risk, or if you like, risk of dying from complications of these diseases. The tablets taken have been shown to reduce the risk of these complications, such as heart attacks or strokes. A very large study, or combination of studies, was published in the *British Medical Journal* in 2013 looking at another option for these diseases. No prize for guessing what this was: exercise. They looked at 16 other large studies investigating the role of exercise compared to medication in treating these conditions. They found that the benefits of exercise and drugs your doctor prescribes were similar in terms of reducing your mortality from these conditions. Particular reference was made to stroke, heart disease, heart failure and prevention of diabetes. Now the cost to society of the medications used to treat these conditions in the Western world alone is probably in the region of trillions of dollars. How many walking tracks, cycling tracks or gyms could you build with this kind of money? How many starving people could you feed? It is likely that the same effect could be shown for weight loss, it is just that we cannot get people to lose weight to do the study, and in these studies they were looking at exercise. Wouldn't you rather exercise than take tablets for the rest of your life? Why not just go for a walk? It would have the added benefit of helping with weight loss as well. Not very complicated, is it?

---

*Huseyin Naci et al., BMJ 2013; 347: f5577.*

Do you realise all the other potential benefits of sustained weight loss, the silent and personal ones no one talks about? How's your relationship going?

# CHAPTER 3

## Your body's response to attempted weight loss. Why you are your own worst enemy

I T WOULD BE nice if everything in life was simple and you just had to eat less to lose weight, but unfortunately, as you are well aware, this is a not the case. Your body will fight long and hard to maintain what it believes is your ideal body weight, which unfortunately for you, if you are reading this book, is a much higher weight than you would like. We do not understand exactly why your body sets its "ideal" body weight at a certain level, but we are beginning to understand, at least superficially, how it goes about protecting this weight level that it sees as ideal. When you think about evolution and survival of the species it is easy to see why you come with built-in protection mechanisms to minimise weight loss at times of famine. All of your cousins who did not have these mechanisms had a survival disadvantage and have long since died from starvation. Those with the protective mechanisms have survived the periods of lack of food in the past, and forwarded these genes on to you. In other words, this is the reason you and your genes are here today, as opposed to you being found in a fossil from the past.

There are several ways the body protects itself from weight loss, allowing it to defeat you when you try to achieve this. The first of these is actually changing your metabolic rate, or the rate at which you burn your calories, to make sure you get the most out of them and they last longer and consequently you last longer in times of serious food shortage. It would appear to do this at least in part by changing the level of various hormones or chemical messengers in the body. The second line of defence is to increase your appetite, again by numerous chemical messengers that affect the parts of your brain that control your appetite. As a result you become incredibly hungry and will literally eat anything you can get hold of and you will not stop until you are overfull with each meal.

The nett effect of these two issues is that you will almost always rebound when you attempt to lose weight. To make matters even worse, as if this is not bad enough, you are likely to overshoot as previously discussed. Your excessive appetite and overeating will continue until your lean body mass, or if you like your mass without fat, gets back to where it started. The problem for you is that the fat is put back on much more quickly than the muscle and when the muscle mass is back to normal you have much more fat than you started with! In other words you have gained weight, reinforcing the fact that diets don't work! If you are going to attempt weight loss, it must be for good.

Now with respect to the first mechanism, the reduction in your metabolic rate associated with weight loss, there are numerous studies in the literature to support this concept. The reduction in the metabolic rate is much greater than would be expected by the drop in weight alone. This can be shown in any mammal, but is easier to do in rats than people as hungry rats do not complain as much. A 10% loss in body weight in rats is associated with a 15% drop in resting energy expenditure adjusted for their weight. This improved metabolic efficiency seems to persist for long periods of time and is only reversed when the restriction of food intake is removed and the weight regained.

---

*Am J Physiol Regul Integr Comp Physiol 287: R1306–R1315, 2004.*

Our understanding of how the body goes about reducing your metabolic rate is not good at this time. There is some evidence that it is related to the levels of thyroid hormones that are crucial in controlling your metabolic rate, or the rate at which you burn calories at rest. This is particularly the active one we call T3, which may be reduced when you drop weight with dieting and may be important in the tendency for weight rebound again after dieting. It seems to go back to normal once you regain your lost weight and there is even some evidence that it tends to rise when you gain weight, trying to protect you from excessive weight gain.

The second mechanism is likely to be the most important in weight regain and perhaps where your feeling guilty is concerned.

I am referring to appetite here, which results in overeating, the reason for you feeling guilty. The hormones or chemical messengers here are numerous as I have said and come from many different areas in the body. Generally they are made of short chains of the building blocks for proteins, called amino acids. The ones that supress appetite get reduced and the ones that stimulate appetite get raised when you attempt weight loss and the result is what we call hyper-phagia, or you eating very large amounts of food before the "off" signal comes through to stop you. "I'm so hungry I could eat a horse!" This is not far from the truth, particularly if you have eaten those processed foods like "chicken" nuggets: who knows what else they contain? Perhaps you have eaten horse, or are at risk of doing so.

The most important organ for production of these chemicals that influence appetite is the gut, and our understanding of these chemicals is gradually increasing but like many areas of medical research we are still really in our infancy here. If we can harness some of these chemicals or produce others like them to take in a pill, we may very well have a simple solution to obesity, or at least to appetite control, which is really the same thing in the end. We are not there yet. I will mention their names so you can look them up and do some further reading if you would like.

## Ghrelin

Ghrelin is a hormone released from the stomach that stimulates appetite and has been called "the hunger hormone" or the "meal initiator hormone". It gets you eating! If you inject rats or humans with this hormone it is a powerful stimulant of appetite and of food intake. It works on the appetite centres in the brain and it works even better if you inject it directly into the brain, but scientists only do this in rats for obvious reasons. Its effect is short lived after a single dose but if you keep giving it you cause long term appetite stimulation and weight gain. Worse still the weight gain is greater than expected for the increase in appetite so it would appear this hormone also influences your metabolic rate. It has been shown to inhibit your ability to use your energy stores of fat and carbohydrate, or if you like to stop you burning calories, and may partly contribute to weight gain by this mechanism.

Ghrelin levels are low in obese subjects and higher in thin subjects but are markedly elevated in those trying to lose weight with diet or exercise or both. It is probably quite important in maintaining body fat stores and nutritional status. Now if you think a bit laterally, one would consider surgery for obesity, such as sleeve gastrectomy where one removes most of the stomach, working because there is nowhere to put the food. Consequently, this is a restrictive type of operation. If patients want to eat a lot after this surgery they cannot physically do so. That is why we started doing these operations. The reality is however they do not want to eat much either. Now where was ghrelin produced? It is quite likely the weight loss with this type of operation is not primarily because of the restrictive effect but because of the hormonal changes (low Ghrelin) associated with the surgery. Nothing is ever as simple as it seems, especially where medicine and your health is concerned.

So why have we not yet produced a drug based on ghrelin to inhibit it and stop you eating? Well unfortunately obese people are the ones with lower levels of this hormone already, perhaps with the body trying to tell you something. When you start to lose weight with dieting its levels rise, making it a very exciting target for drug therapy. The assumption is that its inhibition may prevent the weight regain following weight loss, so watch this space!

Now as everything has to be balanced to be in harmony, your gut also produces what we call satiety hormones to tell you when you have had enough and when to stop eating.

## Cholecystokinin

The one we have known about for the longest is called cholecystokinin or CCK. For over 35 years we have been aware of its potential for inhibiting food intake. It is produced in the small bowel just after the stomach, called the duodenum and the jejunum. After meals rich in fat and protein its levels rise five times and it acts directly on the brain to inhibit appetite as well as acting on the stomach to stop it from emptying, so if you have had a particularly large meal you have nowhere left to put any more food!

Short term administration of CCK in humans and animals does inhibit food intake but long term administration does not cause significant weight loss, so it is probably not a good target for a magic pill.

## Peptide YY and Glucagon like peptide-1

There are several other chemical messengers that are also important in this balance or harmony in the body, controlling that equation of what goes in and what comes out. They are produced further down the gut, by hormone producing cells called L-cells, mainly in the right side of the colon or large bowel. The first of these is peptide YY or PYY. Like the others mentioned, it has many effects. However, one of these is inhibition of appetite and food intake and it is stimulated by eating meals. Giving this extrinsically however only reduces the size of a meal eaten by about a third, but over a long period this may be important. In animal models impaired release or function is associated with obesity. Unlike several other hormones discussed here, it is not reduced in obesity, and sensitivity of the body to the hormone is not impaired in obesity, making it another potential therapeutic target.

The other hormone produced by these L-cells in the right colon that I want to mention is called glucagon like peptide-1, or GLP-1, and I expect that this little player has a big future and you are likely to hear more about it. Like the other satiety hormones it inhibits appetite but it is also important in control of other components of the metabolic syndrome including type 2 diabetes and drugs with a similar longer term action (Exenatide, trade name

Byetta) are already being used to treat this form of diabetes and may potentiate weight loss. It unfortunately needs to be given by injection before meals, like insulin. In diabetes GLP-1 enhances insulin secretion from the pancreas and has other effects such as lowering blood sugar. As such, it has an insulin sensitising effect. It is not useful clinically because of its short half-life or time in the circulation after one dose. Its levels are reduced in obesity and if it is given by injection it does inhibit food intake in humans and in rats. In the chapter to follow there is a section on a particular type of fibre called inulin type fructans, found in onions and some other vegetables, and this fibre increases levels of a chemical butyrate in the colon, which in turn stimulates the L-cells to produce GLP-1 and this may be of relevance in long term weight loss strategies and diabetes management.

A study in 19 healthy obese subjects where this peptide was injected four times daily 30 minutes before meals resulted in a 15% reduction of food intake per meal and a weight loss of 0.55 kg over the five days of the study. The researchers postulated that this relates to the effect on delayed gastric emptying. However, since the study we have come to understand that this compound also has direct effects on the brain to reduce appetite. If the effect could be maintained long term this may be a very effective medication.

*Erik Näslund, British Journal of Nutrition / Volume 91 / Issue 03 / March 2004, pp 439-446.*

*A Wren, S Bloom, Gut hormones and appetite control, Gastroenterology 2007; 2116-2130.*

I am sure you will be seeing many orally active drugs based on GLP-1 coming on the market in the near future as effective therapies for diabetes and hopefully weight loss.

If you have already fallen asleep because of the detail I am going into here, my apologies. However, there is one more important organ I want to discuss here before we are finished. The organ is fat. Yes, fat is not just a place to store energy in its own right, it is also an organ that secretes hormones that control appetite and energy balance in the body. Fat is called adipose tissue and the hormones it produces are called adipokines. The only one I will discuss here is leptin.

## Leptin

Leptin is derived from the Greek work *leptos* meaning thin, and perhaps you should consider it as the opponent of ghrelin. The same brain cells controlling appetite have receptors for Ghrelin and Leptin. The difference is that when you stimulate the leptin receptors your appetite is inhibited. Like ghrelin, it seems to have effects beyond just effecting appetite, and appears to increase energy expenditure, potentially aiding in weight loss. Generally speaking, the larger you are, the more leptin is produced from this fat, but unfortunately the larger you are the less responsive you appear to be to the effects of leptin. When this compound was discovered everyone involved jumped for joy as they felt that finally a target had been found to treat obesity. All that had to be done now was to produce an orally active form that could be given to stop people eating. Unfortunately it was not that simple and not what they had hoped. Given at very high levels the effect seems to very quickly plateau so more leptin is not necessarily more effective, especially in obese subjects who are more resistant to its effects. In other words, it seems to work by stimulating appetite when levels are low and it makes you feel full or satisfied when its levels rise. They can only rise if you have the fat on board to produce the leptin.

The primary effect of leptin seems to be to protect your fat stores by stimulating appetite when there is not enough fat in your body. Low levels are bad, causing hyper-phagia or over-eating, and the levels quickly normalise again once you achieve the magic ideal weight your body has now inbuilt in you, even if it is higher than you would like. Giving more unfortunately was not a panacea helping with weight loss. Higher levels may even be harmful, as they tend to raise blood pressure, make you retain salt and fluid and possibly cause kidney damage.

What I have discussed here is nowhere near a complete list of the intrinsic mechanisms in your body that are all fighting tooth and nail against you in an attempt to prevent your taking your body below what it now believes is your ideal weight. They will not surrender. They will go on and on and on against you, and this is why you need to be so determined and accept that any changes you make are permanent. The moment you give in, you lose, and you end up where you started or likely a bit heavier still, as previously discussed.

Now I apologise if you feel I have discussed these issues in too much detail and you just want a "quick fix" for weight loss. The point I am trying to make however is that there is at this time no such thing. Weight gain and weight loss are very complicated processes; this is a long term battle, being the rest of your life. The better you understand the processes involved the better armed you will be to deal with them. You may also want to take an interest in new drug development and what is around the corner to make it easier for you. The internet is a very powerful tool. The more interest you take in this whole topic the more dedicated and persistent you are likely to be in your approach to it. This may determine how likely you are to be successful in the long term. Knowledge is power.

# CHAPTER 4

# What goes in, what you should and shouldn't be eating and why

T HIS IS UNQUESTIONABLY the most important issue in any approach to weight loss and you need to have a very good understanding of this section of the book.

Just to dispel myths before we begin, food is food. There is no magical food. Organic or pesticide free food has not been shown to be any better for you than any other food in the supermarket or market, so please don't get distracted with rubbish "super food" or "expensive organic food": it is just an excuse for someone else to take your hard earned money off you. In a study published in the *British Journal of Cancer* (March 2014), a research group based at the University of Oxford looked at this issue with cancer as the outcome rather than weight loss. They followed more than 600,000 women for more than 9 years for 16 common cancers, comparing women who always or mostly ate organic (pesticide free) foods with those eating standard foods. 50,000 women developed cancer in the study period. There was no difference in the incidence of cancer in the two groups excepting a slight increase in the risk of breast cancer in those eating the organic foods, not thought to be statistically significant. This seems an amazing finding as the women consciously eating the organic vegetables were almost certainly doing many other healthy things in addition. The study must have been very well controlled to take these into account in the analysis. What has this got to do with calories? Nothing, I'm afraid, but I just wanted to bring this up to dispel myths, and when discussing "what you should be eating and why" it is clearly relevant. Where calories are concerned I promise you there is absolutely no difference between bananas – or anything else – grown organically or by regular agricultural techniques.

We have discussed dropping the term "dieting", but I will be using the term "diet" to describe what you are eating on a day to day basis. This is to say, it is okay to use the noun not the verb. This chapter is best considered as background basic education and it may be that many of you already know most of it. It is crucially important however that you understand the nutritional value of what you are going to be putting in your mouth in the long term. There will be no more comments about English grammar, however, there will be lots of basic maths, because this whole concept is all about balancing equations. You have to be able to ensure that what goes in, in terms of calories on the left side, balances what comes out on the right side, in terms of calories burnt. If it doesn't, you gain weight. I'm sorry, but if you cannot do the maths you are going to fail. There is no magic here either, just common sense. However, there may be some tricks you can use to make things easier. In this chapter we are only discussing the left hand side of the equation — in other words, "what goes in". If you are to make wise and informed choices, you need to understand what you are putting in your mouth.

As a unit to measure the energy in food, or what goes into the equation, I will use the term "calories", but you may also use kilojoules, simply by multiplying by 4.18. In most civilised countries in the world it is mandated by law that this information is printed on the packaging of processed foods so you can make informed decisions and avoid being "poisoned" by the company selling you the food. Do you think this is too strong a comment? Well, hopefully you remember the metabolic syndrome, which, as discussed already, is by far the most common cause of death in Western society. It includes heart disease, strokes, diabetes, most cancers and numerous other diseases. I say again, there is no such thing as natural causes: you are all going to die from something. Remember the metabolic syndrome is best considered as excessive energy intake on the left side of the equation (going in) or inadequate energy expenditure on the right side (going out). The term I use for the left side of the equation in this condition is "carbohydrate poisoning" and for the right side is an "exercise deficiency state". So, if the company selling you the processed food on the left side of your equation unbalances the equation and gives you too many calories, and you do not understand how to check these, you are still going to die younger. When you are dead you are dead, it is a bit academic if you think my using the term "poisoned" is a bit strong. You will not be able to argue from the grave. You would be wrong anyway, you were poisoned!

I would like to stress again, to most people, death is a relatively important issue and understanding how to avoid it may be useful, particularly if you want to remain in the land of the living. We are playing for keeps. If you don't address these issues now, you may not get another chance.

We divide foods into three main groups, which are termed macronutrients, as we take all of them in large amounts. These, as I am sure you know, are carbohydrates, proteins and fats. I would like to discuss each in turn and then discuss how they are put together, which in itself is as important as the individual pieces. This issue relates to food processing or production of what are now termed "ultra-processed foods".

## Carbohydrate

Carbohydrates are the primary energy source that run most of the energy consuming processes in your body. Some tissues can burn either carbohydrate or fat, such as muscle. Some can only burn carbohydrates, such as your brain, with which you are interpreting this information. If the carbohydrate level in your blood, or blood glucose, falls too low, your brain stops working and you will lose consciousness and go into a so called hypoglycaemic coma, from which you die if it is not corrected. This is primarily a concern if you are a diabetic using insulin and accidentally use too much. The rest of us are protected by multiple safety mechanisms built into our body and true hypoglycaemia is very rare.

Now carbohydrate comes in very many forms and they all have around the same potential energy level of four calories per gram. There are only three building blocks that make up all carbohydrates. These building blocks are called saccharides or sugars. The mono-saccharides, glucose, fructose and galactose, are the basic building blocks. All other carbohydrates are made up of combinations of these. Giving just a few examples, sucrose or cane sugar is glucose bonded to fructose; lactose or milk sugar is galactose bonded to glucose; maltose, the sugar in malt, is glucose bonded to glucose. The fibre in your diet, found in fruits, vegetables and grains, are made up of very long chains of these building blocks, which generally we are unable to metabolise ourselves and which literally go straight through us – or would do so were it not for the bacteria in our large bowel, which may partially digest some of them. If the carbohydrate has only one or two of the building blocks it is termed a sugar. *Mono*-saccharide means *one* and *di*-saccharide means *two* of the building blocks, as in some of the above examples. If it has three to nine building blocks it is termed an oligo-saccharide, if more than nine a poly-saccharide, and so on.

For all of these carbohydrates, excepting the mono-saccharides or single component sugars that are absorbed directly by the gut, you need to have the right machinery to break them down into their individual building blocks to absorb them and use them in your body. For example, for the milk sugar lactose, you need the enzyme lactase, and if you don't have it, as is the case with most adults in this world, you will be "lactose intolerant".

In other words, if you drink a litre of milk you will get diarrhoea and colicky abdominal pain, but I am sure many of you already know this. As mentioned before, the fibre in your diet is a carbohydrate you cannot absorb yourself. However, it is still very important as it influences the type and numbers of bacteria in your gut, some of which are good and some of which are bad for you. These bacteria influence your body in numerous ways we are only just beginning to understand in the medical arena.

Now carbohydrates are extremely important in health and disease. In particular, obesity in modern society is strongly linked to carbohydrates. They are likely to be very much more important than fat in your diet, for example, if you are struggling with your weight.

Your body is able to break different carbohydrates down into their individual building blocks at different rates, and how quickly it can do this determines how quickly they can be absorbed. When they are absorbed by your gut they very rapidly end up in your blood stream and have to be controlled there as they are toxic to the body in high levels – as, for example, in diabetes, where the blood sugar is persistently too high. The most important chemical messenger used by the body to bring them down again is insulin, produced by the pancreas. Insulin moves the glucose out of the blood stream and into cells, mainly fat and muscle cells, where the glucose is processed and stored, very often as fat.

We use the term *glycaemic index* (GI) to try to quantify mathematically how quickly the glucose in the blood stream is absorbed from the gut and rises after eating food. The fastest thing to raise the blood glucose, as one might expect, is pure glucose, as it does not have to be processed and we give this a value of 100. A soft drink would be a good example of a very high GI food source, but some fruit juices are surprisingly even worse. Everything else gets compared to this. For example, lentils are more slowly processed and get a level of 40. Low is said to be less than 55, medium is 56-69 and high is greater than 70. Generally speaking, the more refined food is, the more quickly it is absorbed, but some starchy foods like potatoes are also rapidly broken down and absorbed. If for example one is looking at potatoes, white bread and white rice, the body is unfortunately very good at breaking these down and their glycaemic index is high or very close to 100.

Well what's the problem? There is no point in wasting time, is there? I would have to confess generally that is my approach to life, as all my friends know, but this is likely to be the wrong approach here. Let us consider car-bohydrate as being like a car – the type with wheels, I mean. If you are the occupant of a car that crashes into a tree at 100 kilometres per hour, it makes a terrible mess of you and the tree! If it hits the tree at 10-20 kilometres per hour, you may only get a bruise or two. Your body and the GI index are much the same. When something with a GI index of 100 hits your body it causes a very rapid spike in the glucose level in your blood followed by a very rapid and high spike in insulin secreted into the blood stream to try and control the rise in the level of glucose. This is not a good thing.

An alternative way of looking at this issue is to imagine a small sink with a small plug hole, where the water going down the plug hole is running at the maximum rate, equivalent to the maximum rate your body can metabolise the glucose load usefully and healthily. If you pour the water out of a jug slowly into the sink it all goes down the plug hole and disappears. If you walk up with a 20 litre bucket and tip it suddenly into the sink, very little goes down the plug hole and most goes onto the floor! The bucket approach is to the body like eating high glycaemic index foods or drinks. That's right: I am talking about the can of coke or fruit juice you had with your lunch!

Now which tissue in the body takes the most of the overflow glucose (or water which would have ended up on the floor in the above example) in this dire situation of potential glucose (sugar) overload? That would have to be fat, wouldn't it? Thank goodness the floor didn't get wet! Fat cells are experts at this when called to duty in just such an emergency situation. They soak up all the excess in a jiffy. As a result a very large proportion of the glucose or carbohydrate you have just ingested is shunted rapidly into fat cells. No other cells can take in so much in such a hurry; they are like the small plug hole in the sink. What do the fat cells do with it? Well, that is easy: they turn it into more fat, lucky you! More fat just in case a "rainy day" comes up and you need to use it as you cannot get out to eat (or to hunt and gather food as your ancestors did in the past). Pity you are living in a place where it "never rains", isn't it?

Now, as I mentioned before, your body is constantly using glucose to power your brain, your heart, your muscles, your liver and many other types of cells. If you absorb the carbohydrate slowly, as would be the case if you had the lentil soup, instead of the white bread, potatoes and the soft drink for lunch, it would have moved gradually and preferentially into these tissues and be burnt and gone forever, just like the water going down the plug hole!

Now when it seems bad enough that we are already eating refined foods with a high glycaemic index, there may be another serious issue apart from simply getting fatter. It is believed that with repeated high spikes in insulin and glucose after meals, the insulin receptor which the insulin acts on may become down regulated or less sensitive (worn out) to the actions of the insulin. This means you need higher levels of insulin to control the blood sugar. It is a bit like driving a car with worn out brake pads to stop the wheels: you have to push harder on the pedal. This situation is termed insulin resistance or early diabetes. This is the beginning of the metabolic syndrome as described earlier and the consequences as you now know are very serious.

As another example, if one looks at something like white rice consumption in different Asian countries and you graph this against the levels of diabetes in those countries, you get a straight line. The more white rice eaten in a country, the higher the risk of diabetes in that country. The association does not prove one causes the other. However, given the mechanism above it would seem likely they are related.

Is this a big problem? Based on figures in 2010 there were 92.4 million people with diabetes in China, 50.8 million in India and this compares with 26.8 million in the USA, where it is considered a huge and growing problem, in terms of medical resources and financial cost. You be the judge. White rice is only one of numerous offenders in terms of glycaemic index and not likely to be important in the USA. Any fast food giants come to mind here?

*Yang et al., N Engl J Med 2010; 362: 1090-1101.*

Now nothing in life is ever as simple as it seems, as I am sure you are all well aware. The glycaemic index is all about glucose. It is no good for estimating how rapidly fructose is absorbed. If you take in fructose it does have a small effect on the blood glucose level but only just, with it having about the lowest glycaemic index possible of 20, almost off the bottom of the scale. Not really surprising, as glycaemic index just measures glucose not fructose anyway. No point in counting cats if you only have dogs. So it must be good for you, must it not? Well, I'm afraid it is definitely not good for you, at least not in large amounts. In small amounts it seems to help with the metabolism of glucose and does no harm, as occurs if you consume fruits that contain fructose in small amounts. You should not eat huge amounts of sweet fruits as the sugar in these is largely fructose. The problem is that those food processing giants have discovered it and it is even sweeter than sucrose or cane sugar. Unfortunately for us it is also very cheap, coming from sources such as corn syrup, which is about 50%-60% fructose and the rest mainly glucose. So do you remember where food processors put the cheap corn syrup? Well obviously in anything that needs to be sweet and that they can sell to the gullible public such as you. I don't think they give a rat's arse about you, they are only interested in your money, so please hand it over! As a result, soft drinks, sweets, and any processed sweet foods are loaded with the stuff! These are still high GI foods as they usually contain glucose and/or sucrose as well, but also a lot of fructose.

Now fructose is a sneaky little bugger. It does not announce itself with the doorbell and come in through the front door, triggering insulin release and appetite regulating hormones such as its sibling glucose does. It sneaks in the back door and is metabolised very rapidly, much more so than glucose. So what would your body do with excess fructose? Well that's easy, and the same answer keeps coming up: it turns it straight into fat. Now glucose can be metabolised literally all over the body, such as muscle and the brain, to get rid of it. The machinery for metabolising fructose is found almost exclusively in the liver. Your liver cells go into overdrive, converting the sudden huge load of fructose from your sweets and soft drink straight into fat, which is either stored in your liver causing fatty liver or sent into the blood as triglycerides, a type of fat that is soluble in the blood, allowing it to be moved around the body. If the liver tried to keep all this fat to itself it would literally burst, especially if that was a 2 litre bottle of coke you had after working in the yard all morning. The triglyceride levels rise soon after your fructose load is absorbed. These triglycerides are then taken up by your body's fat cells, which swell and become bigger. Lucky you – but wait, there's more! The high triglyceride levels also have added benefits such as causing premature heart disease and strokes. There is also growing evidence that high fructose intake is associated with insulin resistance and diabetes, which follows on logically from the fatty liver already discussed.

The best thing of all is that this happened while you (or if you like your appetite centre) were sitting obliviously watching the TV in the front room of your house and you didn't even see your good old mate fructose sneak around the side and in through the back door. This failure of the body to register fructose's presence may account for the reason there is no "off switch" to tell you that you have had enough of this sugar and partly explain why weight gain is so common in those consuming a high fructose diet. There is also some evidence that fructose consumption reinforces itself: rather than turning off your appetite it tends to increase the desire for sweetness and get you going back for more, and more and more.

If we look at the literature telling us what added sugar in your diet does to your risk of developing cardiovascular (heart and arteries) disease, there is a virtual tidal wave of evidence in the literature that will overwhelm you. It is not a case of does it do you harm – this is beyond question – it is a question of how much harm it does to you. In one of the largest studies, published in the *Journal of the American Medical Association* in 2014, this question was assessed.

They looked at US adults and calculated how much added sugar they had in their diet. They followed the group for 14.6 years, giving 163,039 person years of follow up in total. They enrolled many thousands of people in this carefully conducted study to achieve this. They divided them into four groups from least to greatest amount of sugar consumed. The risk of heart and artery disease was more than doubled between the lowest and highest group. In other words, you double your risk of having a heart attack if you consume a lot of added sugar. This is regardless of race, age, sex, educational level, socioeconomic status, smoking or other risk factors. And the trick here is you don't even have to add it yourself! The makers of all those processed foods you have been eating do it for you at no extra charge to save you the time and effort! Remember how many teaspoons of sugar there are in a can of soft drink or soda, or in those chocolate brownies you were just eating?

You thought you just had to worry about the saturated fat in the bacon and eggs, didn't you?

---

*Quanhe Yang, JAMA Intern Med. 2014; 174(4): 516-524.*

Knowing what you now know about fructose, sugars and what they put in soft drinks and sweets, you would have to be mad to consume them in large amounts, if at all, wouldn't you?

The last of the three primary building blocks of carbohydrate is galactose. This mono-saccharide sugar is quantitatively much less important than the other two as you do not have large food giants trying to shovel it down your throat and it is less abundant in your diet. The usual source is dairy products such as milk, remembering of course that the sugar in milk, lactose, is a combination of glucose bonded to galactose. These two blocks are separated in the gut by the enzyme lactase and each absorbed directly. Like fructose, galactose is metabolised in the liver; however, unlike lactose it is converted to glucose in a three step process that is very rapid. Glucose is a much more stable form of sugar energy in the body and, as discussed already, is used everywhere throughout the body. So from a practical point of view you can view galactose as glucose. Problems really only arise here if there are errors in the enzymatic steps converting the galactose to glucose, such as in the inherited disease galactosaemia where one cannot metabolise galactose and its levels build up. The treatment is simple: avoid milk and dairy if you have this disease.

So you see it matters not only how much carbohydrate you eat, but also what type of carbohydrate you eat. The glycaemic index or GI is now being printed on the nutritional information part of the packet of many processed foods so you can hopefully make an informed choice. Please remember however that the GI of a food is not the whole story as it does not measure the fructose and the processor selling the food does not put a "fructose warning" on the package. Why would they? They are trying to get you to buy it! The fructose is probably even more harmful than the glucose measured by the GI on the package. Look for "sweetened with corn syrup" as well as the GI. In general, however, my repetitive message will be the same: "Stay away from highly processed foods!" This is for many other reasons apart from simply the GI rating. Their appallingly low nutritional value would be one factor and that they may contain large amounts of fructose as a sweetener is another.

When we are discussing carbohydrates not all are directly absorbed as they pass through your small intestine. The small intestine is the part of your gut that absorbs most things that are absorbed from your diet. For this type of carbohydrate we often use the term "fibre", which is made up of long chains of the three building blocks described. You do not have the machinery to break these long chains down into their individual links or mono-saccharides. There are numerous different types of fibre, some soluble in water and some not. Examples would be wheat bran, rice bran, psyllium husks, often they are the outer coating of a seed or the protective layer. One of these needs special mention and you should consider increasing the level of this in your diet. These are inulin type fructans (long chains of fructose) and oligo-fructose (3-9 fructose units in a chain). These are not the same as individual fructose molecules described above. Like all forms of fibre, these effect you indirectly as they are primarily prebiotics or food for the bacteria in your bowel rather than being directly food for you. You cannot really separate yourself from the bacteria in your bowel. They are part of you and have been ever since animals evolved on the planet over hundreds of millions of years. Most of what you pass out of your bowel by dry weight is bacteria: they have consumed most of the food residue that you leave behind, after it passes through the small bowel into the large bowel. There are about 1000-1200 different species or types of bacteria making up about 99% of the bacteria found in the human bowel. You as an individual, will have about 150-200 of these species in your bowel. They number ten to the power of fourteen, or if you prefer one with fourteen zeros after it, a number which is almost too big to imagine. Most of them we cannot culture and we have almost no idea about what they do.

---

*A human gut microbial gene catalogue established by metagenomic sequencing. Nature 2010; 464:59-65*

They outnumber you 10 to 1 in terms of bacteria to human cells, or 25 to 1 in terms of the number of different genes in their DNA compared to yours. They have numerous very important functions you have not even dreamed of. They can even "talk" to you, but you do not need your ears to hear them. We are only in our infancy in working this out and as yet know a lot less than the "tip of the iceberg" but are gradually learning more. The more we learn, the more important we realise they are in health and disease, including obesity. This "gut community" living inside of you can be influenced by many things, including your genes, the type of foods you eat, which includes prebiotic carbohydrate, antibiotics taken during your lifetime, probiotics (live bacteria in capsules or food stuffs like yogurt), and how clean your environment is. It may not necessarily be that the cleaner the better.

Some of the things we do know include the fact that the more types of bacteria there are in the bowel the healthier we are likely to be, from many points of view, including inflammatory, metabolic and autoimmune diseases. These include diseases like obesity, type two diabetes, fatty liver disease, heart disease, bowel cancer, autism, allergies, ulcerative colitis and Crohn's disease, to mention only a few. That's right, you read it correctly: obese people, and other obese mammals, seem to have a different pattern of bacteria or "gut community" in the colon when compared to thin people. Obese people tend to have fewer species and different types of bacteria in their bowel when compared to thin people.

The pattern of bacteria in the bowel in obesity also seems to be associated with long term low grade inflammation in the body, as in many of the diseases above. The patterns associated with health and being thin seem generally not to be associated with this low grade inflammation. This is possibly related to the junctions or joins between cells in the lining of the bowel not being as tight as they should be and as a result you have a relatively "leaky" gut lining. Alternatively, it may be because some bacteria seem to be associated with a thinner protective layer of mucous over the bowel surface cells. This mucous layer shields the cells of the gut lining from toxins or poisons produced by the bacteria in the bowel, predisposing to leakage of these toxins through the gut cell lining into the blood stream. Bacterial products, such as something called lipopolysaccharides (LPS), which are part of the gram negative bacterial cell walls, can then be detected in the blood in higher levels. The level of these lipopolysaccharides in the blood stream correlates with the level of low grade inflammation in the body. The low grade inflammation correlates with obesity and the diseases that accompany obesity.

So we appear to have the age old issue of "good versus evil", even when we are discussing some difficult issues such as the makeup of the bacteria in your bowel. Excuse the pun, but this is very important shit! The next question is obviously how do we change the balance in favour of good rather than evil? Could we simply change the bacteria in your bowel with the result being you managing to effortlessly lose weight? Well, that is a difficult question when we don't really understand much of what we are dealing with, in what direction we need to push, and how to push, let alone how hard to push!

The answer may still be yes, but probably in combination with all the other things discussed in this book if you want the weight loss to be sustained.

A fascinating twin study demonstrates this concept. Using identical twins who were discordant for obesity – in other words, one was thin and one was fat – the importance of the type of bugs in the bowel was proven. Identical twins are a good model to use because they have the same genes, removing the impact of genes on the study results. The faecal material of each twin was transplanted into identical mice in a germ free environment. The recipient mice from the fat twin got fat and the recipient mice from the thin twin stayed lean, with statistically less fat than the mice given the alternative faecal transplant. The mice were both on identical low fat high fibre diets and allowed to eat as much as they liked.

*Ridaura et al. Science 6 September 2013: Vol. 341, no. 6150.*

If one looks at the major types or phyla of bacteria in the bowel in an attempt to understand this, some but not all studies in humans suggest that the difference is in the bacteroidetes group compared to the firmicutes, the latter being lower in obesity. It is likely that many types of bacteria or groups of bacteria are important; however, there is one rapidly rising star out of many thousands of possibilities and it seems to be quite important. It has the name Akkermansia muciniphila (AM). Sorry about the long names, but the bacteria tend to come with these. This is present along the gut and makes up 3%-5% of the bacteria in the bowel in healthy thin people and mice. The more you have the lower are many markers of inflammation in the body and the less "leaky" your gut tends to be, possibly because these bacteria tend to thicken the protective mucous layer over the cells in the gut lining. They may also have effects on the metabolism of fat and glucose, leading to weight loss as its abundance correlates inversely with body weight in both mice and humans. Its actions in the gut may inhibit appetite as well.

In a study looking at this issue, fat type 2 diabetic mice on a high fat diet were noted to have a lower level of AM in their bowel than their lean healthy counterparts. Feeding these mice with prebiotics (oligofructose) completely restored the levels of these bacteria to normal, increasing them by 100 times. Remember, prebiotics are just types of carbohydrate that you cannot absorb, but that the bacteria in your bowel can utilise. This was associated with thickening of the protective mucous layer over the cells in the bowel with loss of the evidence of a leaky gut (decreased LPS) and inflammation in their bodies. More importantly, these mice lost fat and lost weight but ate the same number of calories as their fat counterparts, who were on the control diet without the oligofructose.

They also took an alternative approach, directly feeding AM to the mice as opposed to feeding the carbohydrate prebiotic oligofructose. Not only did the mice that were fed these bacteria lose weight and lose fat in their bodies, their diabetes was completely cured. All this with no change in the food or calorific intake! In other words, it somehow stimulated oxidation or breakdown of fat and glucose directly and the mice didn't have to make any effort at all!

These data suggest that these bacteria somehow play a role in the control of fat storage in the body, metabolism in fat and control of blood glucose, preventing diabetes. They are talking to you! How they talk to you and do this is very complicated and outside the scope of this discussion. Read the article if you are interested. It is free on the internet.

*Proceedings of National Academy of Sciences of the USA, Vol. 110, 9066-71, May 2013.*

Pretty amazing stuff!

Now you may say this is not representative, being an artificial high fat model in a mouse, but do you know how much fat there was in the that big mac and fries you just ate! I hope you didn't have the soft drink too!

So if it is all so simple and straightforward why are these therapies not available to people? Well, partly because not enough studies have been done in people to prove they work and partly because we do not want to cause harm. The literature I am discussing is only months old at the time of writing this. The medical literature is littered with "misadventures" where something seemed like a good idea, but when it was done it caused harm, not benefit. For example, the use of vitamin A, like antioxidants, given to prevent lung cancer in smokers because they had lower levels of the anti-oxidants on testing and this was believed to possibly be the cause of the cancer. This study was stopped because far more people taking the antioxidants got cancer than the controls. This study is detailed in a prior publication "Do You Want to Live to Be 100?"

There were 12 probiotic intervention studies in humans look-ing at obesity discussed at the World Congress of Obesity, in Kuala Lumpur in March of 2014. Most used lactobacilli, none used AM, and the results were disappointing at best. A review of 26 randomised controlled trials of prebiotic use in humans did show some mildly positive effects on insulin and glucose levels but results were contradictory between studies and no definite recommendation could be made. These studies were not looking primarily at inulin like fructans, however, and perhaps need to be redone with these.

*British Journal of Nutrition / Volume 111 / Issue 07 / April 2014, pp 1147-1161*

There was one recent study involving inulin type fructans (ITF) in humans, conducted over 3 months with 15 obese women in each group. The two groups were placebo (no treatment) versus ITF supplementation in the second treated group. Eight grams of ITF taken twice daily was used in the treatment group and well tolerated. There was quite a marked statistically significant change in the type of bacteria in the bowel towards more friendly healthy type species. There was however only a minor loss of fat mass in the ITF group compared with the placebo group, which did not reach statistical significance. It is notable that there was no loss of fat mass in the placebo group. One cannot help but wonder if this lack of statistical significance was because it was such a small study group or short study duration and, if either of these were changed, whether the result may have been different. At least the trend was in the right direction and more research needs to be done.

*Gut 2013; 62: 1112-1121.*

I am a bit impatient, and I do think we move too slowly from research labs to offering treatments to patients, especially where potential cures for cancer are concerned. Many of my colleagues and the lawyers working for patients harmed would tend to disagree, however.

In summary, not all carbohydrates are the same. You are not only feeding yourself with these food stuffs, you are feeding the enormous bacterial community that lives within you, which I have shown is very important in health and disease. Our shift from low GI complex carbohydrates to high GI highly processed food is not a good thing. Try to stop eating the highly processed foods: you are likely to benefit for making the change.

The prebiotics or fibre type mentioned here that seems to increase the good bacteria in your bowel, the oligo fructans and inulin type fructans, are found in commercial preparations made from chicory root, and in onions, leeks, garlic and bananas. The down side of this is that they are processed in your gut by bacteria that produce methane gas, with obvious consequences.

Probiotics and prebiotics are not likely to be the whole answer in the war on obesity and should not be regarded as a cure but may be a useful weapon to use in the war, along with exercise and reduced calorific intake, among other things.

## Protein

There is much less controversy with respect to protein types and what we need. We have a much better understanding of this than we do of carbohydrates, but it is probably still a bit like the tip of the iceberg and we have a lot to learn. Protein is essential for growth and development and for maintenance of your body. Things like your hair, nails, skin and muscles are made almost completely of protein. From a calorific point of view protein has the same energy level as carbohydrate, with roughly four calories per gram of protein.

The building blocks used to construct proteins are called amino acids. There are 20 of these used in constructing our body (some feel there are 21). Nine of these are said to be essential amino acids in that we cannot make them ourselves and rely on intake from the diet to supply them. Generally speaking, there are amino acids in almost all foods, but sources of animal protein tend to be more complete than plant protein sources with respect to the essential amino acids. The exceptions to this are soy and quinoa protein, which contains all essential amino acids. If you are avoiding animal protein sources you need to combine various plant sources to cover all the essential amino acids groups and you need to do some reading to educate yourself here. All will be covered if your diet includes any of the following: meats, eggs, dairy products, soy, quinoa or fish/seafood. Foods such as rice, wheat and other grains, legumes, nuts and seeds contain some but not all of the essential amino acids, so they need to be eaten in combinations. Unlike carbohydrate and fat you cannot store protein, and any that is unused is metabolised and excreted as nitrogen or urea in the urine. The amount you need is dependent on the quality of the protein because you need to get all of the essential amino acids and this is most efficiently eaten as a small amount with each meal rather than one large hit.

Assuming you are eating high quality animal protein you need about 0.75 grams of protein per kg of body weight per day. If you are pregnant or breast feeding then this rises to at least 1 g per kg per day.

Protein is potentially toxic if eaten in very large quantities, as is the case where some weight trainers take 200-400 g of protein per day. The protein is metabolised by the liver and excreted by the kidneys and may strain either of these, but especially the kidneys, particularly if they don't work very well as is the case late in the metabolic syndrome when kidney failure occurs. There is a greater loss of calcium from the body with high protein intake, which may weaken bones, and there is a higher risk of gout as the uric acid that causes gout is a breakdown product of the protein.

There is also some worrying data from animal studies with respect to high protein diets. In one recently published study, 858 mice were fed one of 25 different combinations of protein, fat and carbohydrate over their lifetime and the groups of mice compared. The mice fed the low protein high carbohydrate diet lived the longest and this diet combination was associated with the lowest blood pressure, the lowest blood sugar, the lowest bad cholesterol and the highest good cholesterol. There is also some data from human studies that suggests that diets very high in protein and low in carbohydrate are associated with more heart disease and premature death. The life prolonging effect of the high carbohydrate low protein diet in mice was quite dramatic with mice on the high carbohydrate diet living one and a half times as long as those on the high protein diet. Does this apply to humans? We don't know, but there is cause for concern.

*Cell Metabolism 19, 418–430, March 4, 2014 ª2014 Elsevier Inc.*

## Fat

Fats are a bit more complicated than proteins and carbohydrates in that they are not built out of a finite number of building blocks as are the other two of the three macronutrients. They are no less important and are essential for life. Fats and oils are the same thing, the difference is really just that fat is oil that is solid at room temperature. From an energy or calorie point of view, fat is king, with an energy rating of nine calories per gram.

Fats are made up of fatty acids, usually bonded to a glycerol molecule. They could be thought of as a capital E if you look at the description in Wikipedia online, where the vertical section is the glycerol molecule and the three horizontal lines are the fatty acids. The term "triglyceride" is used to describe this combination.

The type of fatty acid involved determines the type of fat we are discussing. The fatty acids are essentially chains of carbon molecules with hydrogen and oxygen molecules attached. There can be one or two bonds or joins between the carbon molecules in the chain.

*Saturated* fatty acids occur where there are no double bonds in the carbon chain of the fatty acid molecule at all. These potential double bonds between the carbon molecules in the chain have all been taken up or used by hydrogen molecules off the sides. The double bonds are then said to be saturated, or the fat is described as saturated fat. With all the hydrogen molecules sticking off the side of the chains of carbon molecules they tend to stick together and as a consequence are generally solid at room temperature. Animal fats (butter, cheese, lard, ghee) and some vegetable fats (coconut, palm kernel, cotton seed and chocolate) are examples containing saturated fatty acids.

*Mono-unsaturated* fatty acids mean there is only a "mono" or "one" double bond in the whole length of the carbon chain of the fatty acid, which is usually in the range of 13-17 carbon molecules in length. This type of fat is usually intermediate in physical properties, being solid in the fridge or liquid at room temperature as the molecules do not stick together quite as much. Olive oil would be an example of a predominantly mono-unsaturated fat. This group includes avocados, some of the fat in red meat and whole milk products. The types of fats are often mixed.

*Polyunsaturated fatty acids* mean there are "poly" or "many" double bonds in the chain of carbon atoms that make up the fatty acid molecule. As these molecules do not stick together very well they are usually liquid in the fridge and at room temperature. These include most of your familiar vegetable oils but are also found in green leafy vegetables. Nuts and fish contain some polyunsaturated fatty acids.

Now the types of fat mentioned above are natural and generally not harmful, but eating very large amounts of saturated fatty acids may not be good for you. If you eat a lot of any of them you are getting a very dense form of energy, or — if you like — a lot of calories that you need to dispose of somehow. Otherwise, just like carbohydrate you will store them away for a rainy day. You don't even have to turn these ones into fat as they already are fat! Couldn't be easier!

The problems occur, as always, when we start fiddling around with the fats or processing them. Food manufacturers have been doing this for many years, using polyunsaturated vegetable oils primarily and adding hydrogen molecules to the double bonds on either sides of the chain of carbon atoms. As the hydrogen molecules are added "across" the chain they use the term *"trans"*-fatty acids to describe their new creation. This *trans-fatty acid* is solid at room temperature as the molecules stick together and it has a longer shelf life, but most importantly it is cheaper and more convenient for the manufacturer! How do you think they get margarine to be solid at room temperature? What do you think they fry your fish and chips in? Don't be fooled that they said "fried in pure vegetable oil". The vegetable oil was probably trans-fatty acid, especially if you saw it in boxes or cubes on the bench out of the fridge. What type of fat do you think was in the biscuits you got from the supermarket to have with your coffee?! Need I go on?

Now there may be an argument about whether or not saturated fatty acid in natural animal products such as meat is bad for you or not, but there is very little argument about trans-fatty acids. They are strongly linked to an increased risk of cardio-vascular disease – in plain terms, heart attack and stroke. They are also probably linked (some proven only in animal studies) to increased inflammation such as asthma and arthritis, to diabetes and to weight gain, with the fat being placed in the abdomen exacerbating the metabolic syndrome.

So when you think you will be healthy and get fish for dinner, but decide to have it battered and fried for convenience, just remember that it may be ten times as harmful for you as having a fatty steak or roast lamb, dripping in saturated fat. If you have the fish, cook it yourself and use pure unadulterated vegetable oil such as rice bran or peanut oil. Adding just a very small percentage of trans-fat to the fat in your diet may have dire consequences with an increased risk of many of the diseases described above.

Some oils warrant special mention.

*Fish oil* is one of these. It is a freely available supplement and, as the name suggests, it is found in fish, but only some fish. It has no fewer calories than any other oils but its intake seems to protect you from heart disease and possibly some cancers. This effect is specific for cold water fish and the oil comes from the deep ocean phytoplankton all the way up the food chain to these fish and then to you when you eat the fish, or take the oil as a dietary supplement. It does not help you lose weight but may make you live longer.

*Tree nut oil* from eating tree nuts, and possibly peanuts, seems to be similarly protective for cardiovascular disease and for adult onset diabetes when one looks at multiple studies. When one looks at the risk of dying from all causes and the number of times per week you eat nuts, there is a 20% reduction in mortality if you eat nuts every day and it seems the more you eat the greater the reduction in death risk. This so called inverse association is also present for the risk of dying specifically from cancer, heart disease and lung disease. So the bottom line is that not all oils are created equal with respect to health issues. They are all created equal, however, when one is considering calories, at a whopping nine calories per gram, so go easy on them!

---

*Ying Bao et al., The New England Journal of Medicine, November 21, 2013*

At the risk of repeating myself, where you get the oil or fat in your diet from is important, as some are probably better than others, but whatever you do, DO NOT let anyone else mess with your oil or fat before you consume it. Trans-fatty acids are almost certainly very bad for you. You need to understand what they are and be able to recognise them if you are to avoid eating them. If the fat is solid at room temperature, think twice about putting it in your mouth or cooking with it, as it may have been adulterated. This often includes margarine. It likely includes what your chicken and chips were fried in.

There remains a lot of argument about whether or not saturated fat is bad for you, but it is probably not as good as mono-unsaturated or polyunsaturated fats if you review the literature, so try to stick predominantly to the latter two options.

Most of us feel there are three macronutrients that make up the vast majority of the calories we ingest in our daily diet. Unfortunately, not everyone agrees with this and many people feel there are four, not three. The fourth is of course alcohol, or to be more specific ethanol, as to a chemist alcohol means many different compounds, many of which are quite poisonous even in small amounts. Ethanol has seven calories per gram, putting it between carbohydrates and fat in energy level, or fat producing capacity. There is no question alcohol can make you fat and it is quite easy to take in a lot of calories as ethanol without even realising it. Worse still, there is a large amount of sugar hidden with many forms of alcohol consumed and this does not help at all. Have you heard the term beer belly? There are no shortage of these if you look around, particularly at the patrons on the bar stools, or perhaps other family members sitting on the couch in front of the TV "having a cold one and watching the footy". I suppose at least they are exercising one arm holding the coldie and their voice box yelling at the TV, but this is not a very effective strategy for weight loss.

## Processed foods, How to put this all together, Traps to avoid

Now that you are aware of the basic building blocks of a complete diet I expect you feel it should be a simple matter of mixing them together, or getting someone else to do this for you. Sure, it is. There are some very important things to watch out for here and I hope if nothing else I make you more aware of the foods you put in your mouth. There are two separate issues to consider.

The first is the total calorie count of what you are putting in your mouth. The maths is relatively simple, as you know what the calorie value of the carbohydrate, fat and protein making up the food is. Once you start reading labels you are going to be horrified at the amounts of fat and sugars in the foods you are eating. You don't have to be too worried about high protein because that is expensive, so the companies putting this in will put in as little as possible.

The second issue is not the calorie count, it is the detrimental effect on your health of what is going into your food. High glycaemic index food and unhealthy fats are good examples. How toxic is the food to your health?

Before we look at your diet there is one important fact about processed foods that the food processors know but you don't. It is how to mix these food types together to sell them to you and get you coming back, and back and back, with your wallet of course. Let us go back in time, over 100, 000 years in time, and look at how your body and everything in its workings was shaped by evolution or survival of the fittest. It had to learn to cope with everything nature threw at it if it was to pass the genes on to you and not to a fossil in the rocks. You would encounter fat in the form of animal products and sugar in fruits and vegetables. Sugar or sweet things were consumed with gusto if found, but only to a point: there is a limit to how many sweet bananas you can eat before you get sick of them and you stop. Fat was also sought after as an important source of calories but again only to a point where you felt full and the internal mechanisms in your body alerted to stop eating. How much butter can you eat at one sitting with nothing else? Evolution worked these mechanisms out for you tens of thousands of years ago. What your body – and evolution, which shaped and designed your body – never saw was the combination of fat and sugar together. They don't really exist in nature to any significant degree. Consequently, there is no inbuilt mechanism in you to cope with the combination and, unfortunately, whether you are a rat or a person, they are delicious in combination.

If you put rats in a cage with pure sugar, they, like you, eat a little and stop. They do not get fat.

If you put rats in a cage with pure fat, they, like you, eat a little and stop. They do not get fat.

If you put rats in a cage with a processed food combination of fat and sugar, such as cheese cake, ice cream or donuts, which are about 50% fat and sugar, they eat a lot and they get very fat. The "off" switch that should stop them eating seems to be overcome by a very strong reinforcement signal to keep eating because it gives so much pleasure. The combination is like the drug heroin: it keeps you taking it when you do NOT need it for survival of the species. You take the heroin because it gives you pleasure, just like the donuts. You have stepped outside of evolution, it is no longer in control.

The food processors know this and are smiling all the way to the bank. They are the ones in control and they know this as well. To them you are really nothing more than the stupid little rats in the cage! Your diet is being manipulated just like the researchers manipulating the rat's diets in the cage. Why do you think there is sugar in the hamburger buns with your hamburger? Why do you think the fast food giants spend so much time and money sorting out what is the best combination of fat and sugar for their "stupid little rats"? Don't you think it is time you woke up and did something about all this?! How long do you want to live in a cage? How insulting do you find it when someone refers to you as a "stupid little rat"? When are you going to stop eating processed food your body and your mind cannot regulate? You were not designed for processed foods. At the risk of repeating myself, please stop eating them!

I know it is okay, you don't eat junk food, do you? So if you are feeling good about your healthy diet let's look at an example from earlier in the book to get you thinking and I will start with breakfast. Toasted muesli with fruit and nuts, low fat berry yogurt and fresh orange juice. What could be healthier? Sounds good, doesn't it? Well let's look at the muesli packet first. For "toasted" they really mean "deep fried in oil", but that's much the same, isn't it? So the method of preparation makes the muesli 35% fat by weight. Not just any fat, mind you: this is trans- fatty acid made from "healthy" sunflower oil. Well, perhaps before they processed the oil it was healthy! So you get fat proven to cause heart disease and multiply this by nine times to give you the number of calories in the fat. Next is the sugar content and, surprise surprise, it is 15% sugars out of the 50% total carbohydrate. The other component of the total carbohydrate is likely to be more slowly absorbed and is not as harmful. So far, of the muesli's total weight, half is a combination of fat and sugar – the very things you should not be eating.

So what about the yogurt? Well, they may have taken some of the fat out, but if it is sweetened they will have more than made up for it with sugar. Not just any sugar: they go for the cheapest and the sweetest one, corn syrup. This effectively gives you about ten teaspoons of sugar with your yogurt tub dependent on size, and a large dose of fructose into the bargain. At least the fructose will not raise your blood sugar: it will just go quickly and quietly into the liver as fat.

Now surely the freshly squeezed orange juice is okay, isn't it? Well, do you remember the part about glycaemic index in the text above? Rapid rises in blood sugar do many things, all of which are bad for your weight and your health in the long run. One real patient, an insulin dependent diabetic, tells this story, only she was clever enough to work it out for herself. She loves gardening and growing her own oranges and likes to have them for breakfast. If she just eats them there is a slight rise in her blood sugar but within acceptable boundaries. If she juices them her blood sugar goes off the scale and she cannot measure it! "Why?" you ask. She is taking the same amount of sugar and I would agree. The difference is that sugar out of the juice is all absorbed very quickly while the sugar in the eaten orange is trapped in pieces of orange in her stomach and absorbed slowly, and safely, not quickly and harmfully. In reality she also tended to have three oranges when juiced and only one when eaten, as this tended to fill her up the same amount. The same issue applies to any fruit, be it apples or anything else. Do not juice your fruit, eat it! Nature and evolution do not present fruit juice to you, they present fruit, the whole thing. As a general rule do not drink fruit juice of any sort: it has more sugar in it than soft drinks or soda. Eat the fruit and do so in sensible moderation.

Now morning tea comes, so you have a donut or pastry with your coffee? The donut is white flour, fried in trans-fatty acid, rolled in sugar and filled with jam, another word for sugar. The pasty is trans-fat or saturated fat mixed with white flour and sugar and baked, so both are primarily fat and sugar. It is okay, trying to get you in the habit of doing this yourself, looking at yourself and your behaviour critically. I want you to think about everything you put in your mouth and what it is made up of. There are some things you just should not eat or drink and they include things like pastry, biscuits, donuts and fruit juice as a few examples. If you do take these then please make sure it is only on special occasions, never a daily routine. Routines are dangerous, they add up.

I want you to look at what you can do to be more active in your day. Exercise makes you healthy and helps in weight loss but also gives you a possible excuse to avoid situations where you may be expected to eat, just because everyone else is! If you make an effort the results will be impressive! I cannot do it all for you. You need to do it yourself, so start planning and thinking.

# CHAPTER 5

# What comes out, the role of exercise

NOW WHAT MANY of you are not aware or conscious of in the discussion of "what comes out" is that exercise is relatively unimportant, making up a small fraction of energy used from a mathematical view point. That is not to say it is irrelevant in terms of long term weight control, however. As I keep saying, every little bit adds up, especially if it is a habit or routine. Exercise is an important part of a weight loss program or lifestyle change. What people don't realise is that exercise is even more important in preventing the weight regain that occurs with dieting.

Exercise has many benefits apart from weight loss and corrects most of the problems with the metabolic syndrome previously discussed. Your risk of dying from a heart attack for example is more than halved by regular moderate exercise.

If you think you are going to lose weight with exercise alone, you will be disappointed. The small amount of weight loss is quickly corrected by the body's in-built mechanisms to increase appetite and decrease resting metabolic rate. A small amount of food goes a very long way to undoing all that good in terms of cancelling out the potential weight loss you hope to have achieved. You will tend to live longer, however, as the only thing that correlates well with life expectancy is exercise capacity. The number of serious diseases you have and your doctor's opinion count for very little. The type of exercise is not very important in weight loss, but every little bit helps in the big picture, especially if it becomes a habit.

There are many different ways of exercising and I will not review these in detail here. It is part of the overall solution however and needs to be included. Moderate continuous exercise aims to get your heart rate to 70% of the predicted safe maximum. The predicted safe maximum is said to be 220 minus your age, but check with your doctor before you start if you are very obese or have other medical problems, as we may want to reduce your target heart rate a bit. Aerobic interval training is where you train in short bursts, getting your heart rate to 90% of your predicted safe maximum, and there is some evidence that this is more effective in correcting diseases such as the metabolic syndrome, but again check with your doctor to make sure you are not overdoing it here. Physical strength training is also important, where you are aiming to build muscle strength and muscle volume rather than heart and lung fitness. Having more muscle does help you lose fat, which is the primary aim, but you will be disappointed when you step on the scales as muscle is heavier than fat. It is possibly the most effective way of losing fat. This is because you increase you baseline metabolic rate, day and night, twenty four hours per day, those bigger muscles are working for you. They are always hungry and need to be fed, but only while you have them, so keep exercising, they shrink quickly when you stop.

So in terms of what exercise to do, I think you should combine the above options with aerobic training most days of the week but perhaps 1-2 days of weights or physical strength training to have the best of both worlds and get everything going for you.

Most of your energy expenditure during a 24 hour period occurs by your simply "staying alive", and I am not making reference to the Bee Gees here – but jumping around on a disco floor would certainly help a lot of you. There are numerous metabolic and mechanical functions going on in your body when you are awake or asleep and these use large amounts of energy. Your heart has to pump blood around your body and beats more than one hundred thousand times per day to do this. It has to run on something. Did you stop to think how many breaths your breathing muscles need to do in a day to keep you in the land of the living? That would be about 12 per minute, 720 per hour, 17,280 per day. And that is sitting at rest; it would double if you were exercising.

Twenty percent of the oxygen and calories consumed by your body are consumed by your brain, which is an amazing statistic, especially considering the responses you get from some people when you talk to them and the stupid things human beings do. Clearly many of these calories are wasted, in particular by some select groups such as politicians, who at times don't seem to use their brains at all.

It all comes back to being able to balance the equation. Weight gain tends to occur over our lifetimes at a gradual and very slow rate of 1-2 kg per year, or 3-4 grams per day. This may equate to an imbalance in the equation of only 2% per day of energy consumed over energy needed, but it all adds up, gradually and insidiously, and ends up being stored. A small amount of exercise every day may use 3% of your consumed calories and reverse this trend, so you are gradually losing weight, or at least not gaining as quickly, if at all. Something as simple as one apple per day may swing the balance the wrong way. Remember, one apple per day is 365 apples per year. An apple a day does not necessarily keep the doctor away!

So how should you go about increasing your daily exercise in an attempt to balance this equation? Well, you shouldn't have to think very hard about this, because it is very simple, but you do need to actually think and then act, as everyone's situation is different and it will require YOUR input. This is not something someone else can do for you.

*You should consider the issue in terms of:*

A. What you can do differently or incorporate in your usual daily activities or lifestyle.

B. What additional efforts you can make on top of your usual daily activities.

I will make as many suggestions as I can think of in a couple of minutes; you have your whole life to think. Write down what you are planning and do it.

### A. *Things to incorporate in your daily routine.*

-If there is a lift in your building, for goodness sake use the stairs. If this takes too long you will just have to get to work earlier, won't you?

-Walk up the stationary stairs next to the mechanised ones in the shopping centre, airport and railway stations for example.

-If you drive to work, park a block away and walk the rest of the way – and don't drive for short trips, walk!

-If you get public transport, get off the stop before home or work and walk the rest of the way.

-If you sit and watch TV every day, perhaps the news for 30 minutes, replace the couch with an exercise bike or a walking machine and use this for the duration of the show. Obviously you may need headphones or to turn up the volume of the TV.

-If you can safely ride there (work or elsewhere) on a push bike, then do so! Don't take the car!

-If you have room in the yard, get yourself a dog and make sure you take it for a walk EVERY day.

-Get one of those wrist devices they call a pedometer, which measure the number of steps you take in a day and aim to improve. The more the better, but 10,000 would be a good start.

## B. *Things to do in addition to your daily routine. In your "spare time"*

You will need another toy to do this, one that measures your pulse rate. These are available in any sports stores.

-If you say you haven't any spare time you wouldn't be reading this book so make some and stop with the excuses! You will have lots of spare time when you are dead and you will be there sooner with that attitude. May be a bit hard to exercise once you get there, though ...

-Go for a walk every morning or evening or both. The chair in front of the TV will still be there when you get home. You can record your show and watch it later. Preferably do this with a friend, as a group or with your spouse as you are more likely to get out of bed in the morning and go for that walk if you know your friend or neighbour is waiting outside for you to join them. You can't let them down. This is basic psychology.

-Get a gym membership. The more expensive the better: this will make you more likely to go and use it. Remember, it is not only aerobic exercise that is important. If you do weight lifting exercises you will build your muscle bulk. This in turn then works for you, as we have discussed: while you are resting, burning calories as muscle is much more expensive to run, in terms of calories, than fat.

-Get a personal trainer, if you are lucky enough to be able to afford one – then someone else other than me will be telling you to get off your backside.

-Join an exercise group, one that you pay for to make sure you attend. Get fit classes or boot camp classes are very popular and widespread before and after work.

-Buy yourself a bike if there is somewhere safe for you to ride it. Again, the more expensive the better because you will feel all the more guilty if you do not use it!

-Take up a new team sport. It is likely to be helpful socially as well as keeping you fit and your weight down. As part of a team you will have to go to training and the games as you will be letting the rest of the team down if you do not. Again, do not underestimate the psychology of these type of arguments and sign up while you are feeling motivated. It does not have to be sport; it could be a walking or bushwalking group for example.

A lot of this takes courage and sometimes it is easier to do this sort of thing with a friend or partner. I am not trying to give you anything like a complete list, just a few examples for you to build on. The most important thing for you to realise is that, if this is to be effective in the long term goal of weight loss, it has to be a long term habit or if you like a lifestyle change, for good, not for "the season" but for life.

So the next question is how much exercise do you need to do to help in weight loss and to be effective in preventing weight regain?

The answer is quite a lot, and remember, I never said this was going to be easy. Evidence suggests you need 150-250 minutes of moderate intensity physical activity per week to aid weight loss and help prevent weight regain, associated with your changed dietary habits, NOT alone. There is evidence that weight loss and weight maintenance is improved with more than 250 minutes of moderate intensity physical activity. So we are talking of an absolute minimum of 30-50 minutes of exercise per day for five out of 7 days.

---

*American College of Sports Medicine Position Stand, 2009*

Remember there are 168 hours in a week. If you cannot spare 3-4 of these to potentially save yourself from a premature death, then that is your choice. I don't want to hear you complaining to me "I don't have time!" You are the one in control of your life and you are the one to prioritise your time. Like all the other suggestions in this book, no one else is going to do it for you.

# CHAPTER 6

## How to cheat, Tricks to make weight loss easier

S O IF THERE are some tricks we should be using to help lose weight why has it taken doctors so long to tell us about them?! Well, this is because we are only really just discovering them and as yet some of them remain unproven but I will tell you about them anyway because I think they may help.

### *Brown fat*

Brown fat is nothing like the fat you are undoubtedly very familiar with if you are reading this book. The brown fat, or brown adipose tissue (BAT) is stacked full of small things called mitochondria that are the tiny furnaces inside the cells in you which produce energy and which keep you alive. How do they make heat? They burn fat and sugar. Getting interesting, isn't it?

Now BAT has really only been shown to function in adult humans since 2009. Since that time it has been shown to be a flexible tissue that is able to increase its presence and its activity. When you get cold your body has only two mechanisms to increase energy production and warm you up. Your brain will tell you that you are cold and need to look for warmer clothing and get out of the cold, but if you were unable to do so and your body could not make more energy you would die. The usual response to being cold is to begin using your muscles involuntarily with shivering, thus producing heat and warming you up. The alternative option is to turn on the non-shivering form of thermogenesis or heat production, using your brown fat. Now the bad news is that not everyone has brown fat in significant amounts, and the worse news is that the fatter you are the less likely you are to have a useful amount. Your body is not stupid: if you are well insulated you are unlikely to need it any way.

So how do you get it? Well, to induce your BAT you need to get cold. There are several studies in humans, and numerous studies in animals, showing that it is possible to increase both the function and the amount of BAT in your body with exposure to cold. There are also studies showing higher levels of BAT activity in humans during the winter than during the summer. As you induce your BAT your tolerance for the cold and your likelihood of shivering both decrease. Being exposed to 15 degrees Celsius for 6 hours per day for 10 days shows measurable changes in both volume and activity of brown fat. Sound a bit dramatic? Well not really if you think about it. Where do many of you spend more than 6 hours per day? The answer is indoors, be it at home or at work. You cannot do anything about the temperature outside anyway, but you can reduce your clothing. The implication here is if you spend your time in a cooler environment you may increase the amount and the activity of your brown fat, with potential implications for your weight because brown fat is very good at burning calories and you didn't even have to do any exercise at all! Now if you run off looking for warmer clothes to wear in your cooler environment you are clearly wasting your time, and potentially electricity if you are using an air conditioner to cool the room down inside.

Now that you know brown fat exists, and you have cooled your environment down to get yours to grow, the next obvious question is how do you switch it on and get it to burn calories? Not only does it help you lose weight, it also lowers your blood sugar, reduces insulin resistance and lowers blood fat levels. If it had a simple on-off button I'm sure you would have worn this out long ago. There are multiple messengers in the body that control the activity of your brown fat and we are only just beginning to understand a few things about them. They include feeling cold as discussed and thyroid hormone which increases the body's metabolic rate and energy expenditure, partly at least via its effect on your BAT. Your BAT also becomes active and increases activity after meals, particularly higher protein meals, burning calories but not enough to make up for the whole meal and negate its effect on your weight.

So what we really need is a trick to turn on your BAT and make it burn your fat.

It might sound too good to be true but nature does provide a few of these and it may not be long before we copy these to make effective drugs to increase your metabolic rate and help you lose weight. One of these is capsaicin or the active ingredient in chilli peppers that makes them feel hot. This has been shown to increase BAT activity and burn fat in rats with resultant weight loss. It has also been shown to increase thermogenesis or heat production in humans, but as it is hard to get people to ingest large amounts, for obvious reasons, it is harder to show any significant effect on weight loss. Capsaicin doesn't really burn you, it just activates a receptor in the lining of your mouth and elsewhere to make you think you are being burnt, there is no damage to the lining of your mouth or any other part of your gut. Activation of this chilli receptor still hurts however and the good news is there are similar compounds in sweet red peppers (CH-19 sweet or capsicum anuum), called capsinoids, which are nothing like as hot as capsaicin on either end of your gut. The capsinoids have similar effects on BAT with resultant heat production and fat burning effects shown in both small rodents and humans in multiple studies. The problem is that they only seem to work if you have the brown fat for them to work on, or the chilli receptors (studies in mice only).

In one study in Japan, 18 men were given these capsinoids to assess the effect on their BAT. They wore light clothing at 19 degrees Celsius for 2 hours beforehand and had a special scan (FDG-PET) to check if they had any active brown fat in their body. Ten had active brown fat and eight didn't. They were then given 9 mg of capsinoids by mouth and had tests performed at a more comfortable temperature of 27 degrees for 2 hours. The group with the brown fat showed increased energy expenditure of 15.2 kilojoules per hour with the capsinoids having no effect on the group without the brown fat. The placebo medication had no effect on either group. Weight loss was not measured as the study only went for 2 hours after ingestion of the capsinoids. However, weight loss has been demonstrated in rats studied for longer periods, and humans are similar to rats in many ways, as I keep telling you!

A year later the same author looked at the effect of daily oral ingestion of capsinoids 9 mg for 6 weeks compared with placebo. After the 6 weeks there was a significant increase in cold induced thermogenesis (indicating increased brown fat activity) in the treated group but no increase in the placebo group over the initial level. The whole body energy expenditure rose by about 200 kcal per day for a 70 kg male, quite a significant jump over the long term, in terms of potential for weight loss. Another group has shown a statistically significant drop in visceral (intra-abdominal) fat over 12 weeks of capsinoids 6 mg per day but no significant weight loss overall, although weight did drop slightly in the treated group.

Capsinoids are not absorbed from the gastrointestinal tract, they work, as discussed, on the chilli receptor in the lining of the gut (TRPV1) and stimulate a part of your nervous system called the sympathetic nervous system in the brain.

This nervous system then signals to white fatty tissue to break down fat (lipolysis) and release it into the circulation, and also to the brown fatty tissue to take this free fat out of the circulation and burn (oxidise) the fat to produce heat. The capsinoids stimulating this part of the nervous system would leave doctors worrying that the capsinoids may increase the blood pressure, as this is a function of the sympathetic nervous system also. However, there is no effect on systolic or diastolic blood pressure at doses of 15 or 30 mg daily and there were no other discernible side effects either.

*Am J Clin Nutr 2012; 95: 845–50, J Clin Invest, 2013, Am J Clin Nutr, 2009, Int J Toxicology 2009.*

The Japanese researchers also looked at an extract from the seed of a plant called Grains of Paradise. This is related to the plant ginger. The active ingredient in this 6-paradol is known to activate BAT and increase energy production in small rodents. The study was similar to the one above in terms of design and methods. Twelve out of 19 men were positive for BAT and only this group responded to the GP extract, with a significant increase in energy expenditure within 2 hours of taking the extract, similar to the effect of capsinoids. There are likely to be many other natural substances out there that activate brown fat and increase fat burning or energy expenditure.

*Br J Nutr. 2013 Aug; 110(4): 733-8.*

The problem with brown fat is that the ones who really need it for weight loss are obese people and they have much less of it than lean people, making it less useful as a target to induce weight loss. We need other tricks apart from cooling people down to turn it on, making it potentially more useful in this battle with obesity. Capsinoids are a good start. It would be great if we could turn white fat into brown fat, wouldn't it? It is very early days; however, there is some suggestion that the drug sildenafil may be able to do this, at least partially, and as yet only in mice. It has been shown to increase brown adipose fat activity by more than 400% in mouse studies. It is apparently quite useful for obese mice. You may be familiar with this drug by another name, Viagra. It apparently has other uses not strictly related to fat mice.

*April 2013 The FASEB Journal vol. 27 no. 4 1621-1630.*

### Cocoa

Surely eating chocolate doesn't make you lose weight, I thought it made you gain weight? Well there is chocolate and there is chocolate. If you think we are talking about so called "milk chocolate" then you are sadly mistaken. There is hardly any cocoa in milk chocolate and you are quite right it does make you put on weight. Loads of weight, in fact, because it is just fat and sugar anyway, as usual in a 50/50 mix. You would be hard pressed to find anything with more calories.

I am talking about cocoa which gives chocolate its flavour. Pure cocoa extract is bitter and does not contain fat. It does however contain many antioxidant chemicals called polyphenols. These include the phenolic acids and flavonoids, to be more specific, but the names are not important. What is important is that these substances seem to have many properties that I think are potentially going to be very important in our fight against obesity. They have been shown to have many effects including weight and fat loss in animal models and to reduce blood fats. In a study presented at the World Congress of Obesity in Kuala Lumpur in 2014 the effect was looked at in high fat diet induced obesity in rats. In the group of rats fed a high fat diet, the addition of cocoa extract to the diet over 12 weeks resulted in weight loss, reduction in visceral fat and blood fats when compared to the group of rats fed the high fat diet without the cocoa. On further detailed investigation, the microscopic machinery for burning fat was increased or "turned up" and the microscopic machinery for making fat was "turned down" in the rats fed cocoa. This finding is in line with other research in numerous studies over the last 10 years or more showing that something in the cocoa enhances thermogenesis or fat burning and inhibits fat production.

*Nutrition Volume 21, Issue 5, May 2005, Pages 594–601.*

There seems to be less in the literature about dark chocolate inhibiting appetite; however, I feel it is effective in this regard. There are some studies looking at dark and mild chocolate showing that dark chocolate is better at supressing appetite, causing one to feel full and reducing subsequent calorie intake. The reduction in the calorie intake was quite impressively 17% lower after the dark chocolate.

*Nutrition and Diabetes (2011)*

At the time of writing this there was a lot in the scientific literature about rats and cocoa but there were no good studies I could find looking at human beings and the appetite suppressing effects of pure cocoa. This being the case, I had to do my own study, but as I didn't have any rats I had to make the most of the next best thing I could find, my overweight medical colleagues. There are a number of them who work with me, predominantly giving anaesthesia for procedures I perform, and as part of the deal I had to provide lunch. Well, on this occasion I had a surprise for them! I had found a capsule making machine on the internet and made capsules filled with processed cocoa powder, the simple type you put in your chocolate cake mix. Instead of their usual curry and rice they were presented with cocoa capsules. I had no idea how much to give them so we guessed at ten capsules and I took them as well, all in the name of science. They were taken on an empty stomach with water or coffee. Now admittedly there were only eight participants in this trial and it was not blinded. However, seven of the eight found the cocoa to be markedly effective and did not feel hungry at all for the rest of the day, even though they had not eaten since breakfast. One of the doctors could not even eat any of his evening meal as he felt so full, despite the fact it was a special occasion and his partner had gone to great lengths preparing it! The single failure in this study has the real name Martin, and he was caught stealing biscuits and cheese from the patients in the mid-afternoon and he was shamed appropriately. This clearly does not prove anything as the study has many potential problems in interpreting the results. However, I have little doubt that processed cocoa powder taken on an empty stomach is a good appetite suppressant and the effect lasts for many hours. Ten capsules is about two heaped teaspoons or one rounded tablespoon, taken with water on an EMPTY stomach. You will have to be quite determined trying to stir it up in the water before you swallow it. It may make you feel slightly nauseated initially as it did me. However, this is a small price to pay if it allows you to go without lunch, with a likely dramatic effect on your weight if you keep it up long term. Interestingly, none of the subjects felt particular hungry that evening and they said they ate no more than usual for the evening meal. What have you got to lose? Try it! It works in rats and their cousins, overweight doctors (in one uncontrolled unblinded study, which doesn't prove its efficacy but I think you will find it useful).

The cocoa has many other potential health benefits including reducing your blood pressure and possibly your risk of heart disease. It is potentially toxic if you take very large amounts, of over 150 g in a day. However, this is a very large amount and if you stick with your teaspoon or capsules you should be okay. Beware that it does contain theobromine, a compound similar in structure and effect to caffeine. This will wake you up and may make you feel agitated if you have taken too much. I was surprised how energised and awake I felt. I certainly did not go looking for more coffee as I usually do in the afternoons.

As most of you are aware there are numerous natural herbs and other plant extracts out there that are aggressively marketed to make you think they are the answer and will, all on their own, be the solution to your weight problem. None of the suggestions I have discussed above are put there to make you think this, but if some are marginally effective, and are combined with many other strategies, they may be helpful. They are not a cure. The people marketing them as a cure are interested in one thing, your money. They have no real interest in your health. You need to assess the evidence and that is why I try to quote studies where I can to back up claims.

A useful example here is the plant extract from Garcinia cambogia. This is a small green pumpkin like vegetable used in Asian cooking for its sour flavour. The skin contains a compound, hydroxycitric acid, which is said to have effects on appetite and production of fat that may help you lose weight. It is suggested that this be taken before meals. In some effects it is a bit like cocoa, where it raises serotonin levels in the brain that may impair appetite. There are many studies in rats showing that it is effective in weight loss, so if you are a rat it looks very promising. In humans however there are a number of studies, some showing a very small amount of weight loss, some showing no effect and others showing placebo (dummy pills) to be more effective than the Garcinia cambogia extract. It is stated to be the secret ingredient in Oprah's weight loss but statements like this do not prove anything so don't be fooled. Only properly conducted scientific studies give you anything like evidence and even these are far from perfect. I am not saying this does not work, just that if it does the effect is probably minimal and it should be combined with other strategies. As far as I can find in the literature it does not do you any serious harm. At the risk of sounding repetitive, this is not the case when discussing some other "natural" therapies such as many herbal therapies to inhibit appetite or increase metabolism. We now have hundreds of Chinese and other herbal extracts that are linked to severe liver inflammation and liver failure. In my line of work I have seen patients die from liver failure or be saved only by a liver transplant after taking these "harmless natural therapies". It may well be we will find some that are helpful but please, proceed with caution and do not be so gullible as to believe everything you read, especially in the context of advertising. Just because you want it to work does not mean it will work, but it does make you very easy prey for those who want your money.

So if you cannot trust the naturopaths, and in my experience you very often cannot, then perhaps the regular scientific medical establishment has something to offer to make it easier to lose weight. Well I am afraid we are not much better, at least in the longer term when it comes to "magic pills" to deal with obesity. There have been a number of these pills marketed, presumably for the same reasons the natural ones are, that being money. The huge pharmaceutical companies have lots of expenses and "money makes the world go around", doesn't it? I may sound a bit sarcastic here but the problem is that when patients and doctors are desperate for a medicine to help a problem like obesity there is a lot of money to be made by the pharmaceutical companies, and they know it. Things get rushed through, perhaps before we have adequate insight into side effects. History often is the best way of demonstrating this. The repeated pattern here has been to release a new drug to the market with great fanfare and promise, only to have the side effects later recognised and the drug withdrawn, the difference being that it is withdrawn by its maker as quietly as possible.

*Fenfluramine*, an appetite suppressant, was one of these. Introduced with great promise it was later withdrawn in 1997 because — oops! — it may cause permanent damage to your heart valves, possibly resulting in death. Sorry about that but if this occurs it certainly helps with weight loss!

*Sibutramine* was another centrally acting (on the brain) appetite suppressant that came out with great promise. Its trade name in Australia was Reductil. It was withdrawn in 2010 when a study noted that obese patients taking this drug seemed to be at higher risk of suffering heart attacks and strokes than those trying to lose weight by exercise and diet alone.

Those currently available depend on which country you live in. In Australia we have two currently licenced for weight loss.

*Phentermine* is one of these, going by the brand name "Duromine". There is no question this is partially effective in its aim of appetite suppression. However, if you look it up on the "my doctor" web-site you will find:

> *Phentermine* should not be used in people with high blood pressure, an overactive thyroid gland, epilepsy, a history of a psychiatric disorder, or a history of drug or alcohol abuse or dependency. This medicine is also not suitable for pregnant women.
>
> Adverse effects include dry mouth, headaches, insomnia, restlessness, nervousness, agitation, fast heartbeat and, rarely, psychosis and hallucinations.

Is it really worth the risk? It does raise you blood pressure and this is one way to potentially shorten your life. It has chemical similarities to Fenfluramine with which it was first released and who knows what is around the corner in terms of side effects yet to be documented.

The second drug available is called *Orlistat* and has the trade name in Australia of Xenical. This drug works very differently and is potentially safer. It inhibits the enzyme lipase produced by the pancreas and which is needed to absorb fat from your intestine. Over periods of up to two years it has been shown in studies to be 3-4% more effective than diet alone. Was that 3-4%? Impressive stuff!

---

*Spotlight on Orlistat in the management of patients with obesity. Treat Endocrinol 2005; 127-9.*

Now the only problem with you not absorbing part of the fat in your diet is that it has to go somewhere and that somewhere is out the other end of you. The result is impressive diarrhoea with urgency to get to the toilet, fatty leakage from your bottom and difficulty flushing your bowel motions as they are so good at floating with all that fat in them! These impressive gastro-intestinal symptoms, which patients quickly link to fat in the diet, tend to make people avoid fat in their diet. As a result, any weight loss may well be because of this avoidance behaviour and nothing to do with the malabsorption induced by the drug. Simpler just to avoid the fat I would have thought. The other issue with this medication is that it causes malabsorption of fat soluble vitamins, Vitamin A, D, E and K, with the potential for deficiency of these.

So it would seem you have your choice of higher blood pressure and a racing heart putting you at risk of a stroke or heart attack, or diarrhoea, abdominal cramps with possible faecal incontinence, or avoid the medications altogether and use other methods. You make your choice.

The other issue for these medications is that they are only recommended for use for 12 months or at most 2 years! Nothing to do with the horrendous side effects, I am sure! Haven't we already discussed why relatively short term interventions are a waste of time when we are trying to achieve a lifelong lifestyle intervention?

# CHAPTER 7

# Food substitution

B Y FOOD SUBSTITUTION I simply mean replacing one food with another, the latter hopefully having lower calories, but if not at least being healthier. Some of the food substitutes have very low calorie content and these are usually fibre type vegetable extracts such as Konjac or inulin that I will discuss in more detail. Most of the options are simply other foods found in your panty or in the fridge/freezer. I will give a short list of examples and tricks you can use to avoid calories. However, the internet is the simplest way of looking for alternatives. For example, why don't you google something like "food substitutes for cream" and see what comes up. This is particularly useful when you are cooking or baking.

## Sugar

I would rather you just kicked the habit instead of looking for substitutes here; however, that is easier said than done. There are numerous chemicals, natural and synthetic out there that can trick the sweet taste buds into thinking they are sugar. They thought they had this sorted 45 years ago when the chemicals cyclamate and saccharin came on the market but then there was semi hysteria in the press that these caused cancer and people shied away from them. I don't know if there was any evidence for this and I suspect this was mis-information from the powerful sugar industry. When you throw enough mud, however, especially with the word *cancer* involved, some of the mud will stick and no one will buy it "just in case".

There are natural alternatives such as Stevia. This has been used in South America for up to 1,500 years. The steviol gly-coside extract from the leaf of this plant is 300 times sweeter than sugar and contains negligible calories. It is generally considered safe and available in the supermarket and online. If you are looking at putting cups of sugar in the chocolate cake mixture you are much better off using something like this. Get the pure extract, however: don't let the food proces-sors mix it with a dozen other things before they sell it to you. You can get small sachets or pills for tea and coffee.

You can use other simple things in your pantry such as va-nilla extract or even unsweetened apple sauce in your baking instead of sugar. Not quite the same but they do the trick and are much healthier

## White Flour

If you must use flour make it whole grain to slow the absorption of glucose. Coconut and almond flour are alternatives. You can even use legumes like black beans or various sorts of peas dried and put through the food processor to replace some or all of the flour in the bread or cakes you are making. That way you get lower calories, slower absorption and more protein to fill you up.

## Fat and Butter and Cream

The easiest substitute here is again pureed vegetables or fruits such as banana, apple, and prunes. If you buy the apple sauce make sure it is unsweetened. You can also use fibre type agents such as inulin, cellulose, maltodextrins and other bulking agents for a similar effect, especially when baking or cooking. There are many different brands with different names so you'll have to read the label. In Australia there are several commercially available types of inulin; *Benefiber* made from wheat and a *Metamucil* brand made from chicory rood extract. These are available in chemists or supermarkets but are quite expensive. It is much cheaper to buy your inulin online but go for the chicory root extract type as this is what has been used in most studies quoted.

## High fat foods, meat and dairy

Well this should be obvious but I will spell it out. Almost all dairy products come in low fat alternatives, but make sure they don't contain extra sugar. This includes milk, yogurt, cream, sour cream and cheese. There is a huge difference in the calories.

Things like sour cream should be substituted with low fat Greek yogurt, as this is likely lower fat than "low fat sour cream", but again, read the label.

With minced beef or sausages hunt out the low fat alternatives if you must have them at all. Minced chicken or turkey breast can be very low fat in your hamburgers or meat sauces.

Read the labels and choose wisely, whether it is salad dressing or peanut butter you are looking at.

## Rice

Rice probably has a lot to answer for in the obesity epidemic, especially in Asia. One of the cleverest alternatives I have seen here is coarsely grated steamed cauliflower, a similar texture for a fraction of the calories. If you must have rice use brown rice to reduce the glycaemic index, or choose something like quinoa that has much more protein and fewer calories. Finely chopped steamed vegetables of any sort will do.

## Mashed potato

Mash something else with fewer calories. Again, cauliflower is a tasty possibility, turnips are another. Much more flavour than potato!

## Floury vegetables like potato and pumpkin

Avoid these if possible and choose some more of the green leafy vegetables

## Spaghetti

Heard of spaghetti squash? If you steam it and scrape out the inside with a fork it looks like spaghetti, with almost no calories. If you must have pasta then as always choose the wholemeal alternative to slow absorption and reduce the collateral damage (to your gut and liver). You can cut zucchini into numerous ribbons to make you think you are eating pasta.

## Potato chips

You shouldn't be even thinking about these. You can make chips out of almost any root or other vegetable. Kale is quite popular. Spray the leaves with minimal oil, put on your salt, chilli powder or whatever and bake until crisp. Alternatives are baked (not fried) beetroot, turnips, carrots or even thinly sliced apple.

## Ice cream

Pureed and frozen banana or frozen yogurt

## Konjac

I mention this as it has almost no calories and is relatively taste-less and can replace things like spaghetti or rice noodles to fill you up. It is a root vegetable native to Japan, southern China and Indonesia. You can make a flour out of the root and in theory use it more widely in cooking but it is very gelatinous or gum like. When used as a bulking agent to fill people up or in sweets it may swell up and if not swallowed property can obstruct the airway or swallowing tube and there have been a number of well publicised deaths associated with candy and jelly snacks. If you take the capsules of the flour to fill you up please swallow them carefully!

## Inulin

This is used, as previously discussed, as a bulking agent in foods by the food processing industry primarily to replace fat. It is one of the few things they put in that does not do you any harm. It may be in your low fat yogurt, for example. It has a similar sort of texture to fat if you mix it with water at the right concentra-tion it will thicken like cream and you can experiment putting it in cakes instead of butter or cream. The down side is the in-creased gas but the upside is more healthy bacteria in the colon and appetite suppression.

## Cocoa powder

I don't really expect you to use this as a food substitute but it is a very good appetite suppressant in my experience. If you get hungry mix a rounded dessert spoon of cocoa with a spoon of inulin and take it as a food alternative with virtually no calories, particularly in the late afternoon, as I will discuss later.

This list is far from complete. I am just trying to get you on track to always look for healthier alternatives to what you are putting in your mouth. If you do it long term it will make a positive contribution to your sustained weight loss.

# CHAPTER 8

## When all else fails. The role of surgery and the options available.

T HE ADVANTAGE OF surgery over non-surgical treatments for obesity is that surgery works and non-surgical treatments often don't. If you have failed to lose weight and have a BMI of 35 or more with other comorbidities such as diabetes then surgery is likely to be effective. The down sides of surgery are that it is very expensive, with the surgeon happy to charge you very large amounts out of pocket, and the fact that things do not always go as planned. The likelihood of dying from the procedure is probably less than 1 in a 100 (between 0.1% and 2% in large studies). However, the likelihood of needing another operation is about 1 in 12, either because the first one does not work as expected with intolerable side effects or lack of weight loss. The surgeons usually have to cut and re-arrange your gut and where they join bits together there may be leaks, which are serious, life threatening and may result in prolonged hospital stays and multiple further interventional procedures. I know because as a gastroenterologist I deal with these patients, quite often performing procedures to try to correct the leaks, and I could tell you some very scary stories. I will refrain however and would suggest that, overall, if you fail to lose weight with conventional methods, you are much more likely to die from medical issues associated with your obesity than surgery for the obesity. I am hopeful that none of this chapter applies to you and we can help you without surgery.

## Options available

In the past there have been a large number of things done to patients with obesity with terrible outcomes. Over recent years surgery is becoming safer and more evidence based in its approach. There are two general ways of dealing with excessive calorie intake from a surgical perspective. You can limit the size of the reservoir where people put their food, a so called restrictive procedure, or you can make sure they don't absorb the food, a so called malabsorption type procedure. The easiest way to do the latter is just to bypass large amounts of the small intestine, the place where we absorb food. That way people can eat as much as they like and it literally goes straight through them. The problem with this is that patients develop many vitamin and mineral deficiencies and they also have a blind loop of intestine left behind that is quickly colonised by bacteria, as it is not regularly flushed out with food. The result of either the blind loop with bacterial overgrowth or the deficiency states causes severe fatty liver disease, then cirrhosis of the liver and death from liver failure, before you even start to worry about all the issues related to deficiencies of multiple vitamins and minerals. Oops, not a good outcome! For this reason intestinal bypass procedures are rarely performed these days. Don't let a surgeon do this type of operation on you.

One of the newer, less invasive techniques that was very popular when it first became available was the laparoscopic gastric band. In this procedure a hollow balloon like band is placed around the upper stomach causing a small reservoir and acting as a restrictive procedure, where you can really only have several mouthfuls of food at a time following the surgery. The advantage is that it is minimally invasive as it is laparoscopic, or keyhole surgery, and it can be adjusted by putting more or less fluid in the band, making it more or less effective. It is also potentially reversible in that it can be removed and normal anatomy restored and there is no cutting, re-routing or removal of any of the gut. The downside is that you can get around its effect by drinking milkshakes or vitamised food all day. Some patients get terrible heartburn or reflux. This is presumably because the upper part of your stomach makes acid, and if it is isolated in a pouch, the acid will run back up your throat as the route the other way is partly obstructed. People tend to stretch the small pouch with time, effectively pulling more stomach through above the band, and they tend to be less effective with time. For these reasons they are starting to go out of favour in Australia.

The next operation to gain popularity in Australia is the sleeve gastrectomy, also called a vertical sleeve gastrectomy, and this is now the most common weight loss procedure in this country. This is also done by a laparoscopic approach where the majority of the stomach is removed, turning it into a tube. This has been likened to reducing the stomach size from that of a football to the size of a banana, reducing its holding capacity from 1500 mls to 200 mls. This is obviously not reversible, and the other 2/3 of the stomach gets thrown in the bucket. This was designed as a restrictive procedure; however, it is likely that there are other things at play here, with loss of chemical messengers produced by the stomach to stimulate appetite such as ghrelin as the patients don't feel hunger as much. When they do eat they can only put about 25% as much food in the stomach as they could in the past and it is not clear whether this or the loss of ghrelin is the most important factor in its efficacy. The problem is that there is a very long part of the stomach that has to be stapled back together to make the tube and if this leaks we have a serious, life threatening situation. Postoperative leaks do not seem to be that uncommon. They are usually effective with loss of 70% of excessive weight over the first 12 months and there is no malabsorption as the route the food passes is not disturbed. Some patients do seem to be able to stretch that banana back towards a football shape, but with resultant weight gain and this is of concern with long term efficacy.

The next most common weight loss surgery performed in Australia is the gastric bypass operation, and this is probably the most common operation in the United States. Here, a bit like the banding procedure, a small pouch of stomach is left at the end of the swallowing tube or oesophagus, as a restrictive procedure. A tube of small intestine called jejunum is then brought up and joined onto this tiny residual stomach. This means that the flow of food bypasses the lower remainder of the stomach and the small bowel immediately after the stomach called the duodenum. The duodenum is where the pancreatic juices and the bile from the liver mix with food as it comes out of the stomach breaking down fat and protein to aid in absorption. Consequently this procedure also results in malabsorption of food, which means you need to be monitored with blood tests and may require supplemental nutrients. It also means there is no stomach or "brake" on food getting to the intestine where it is absorbed, and if you eat very sweet or salty foods you may feel unwell because of something called the dumping syndrome where water moves rapidly into your gut. It is also more invasive, with a longer recovery time and the risk of leaking from staple lines. Like the others, if all goes well, it is likely to be effective in weight loss.

When one compares bariatric surgery to non-surgical treatment for obesity then I'm afraid the surgery comes out on top. One has to remember that you are really comparing people who failed medical options with people having surgery. Those who succeeded with weight loss are already thin and are not in the equation at all, as in some of the real life examples given. I am hoping you will be among the successful, without surgery, when you have followed the suggestions in this book. If you do fail however surgery is effective and requires very little input from you except for the pain and suffering involved.

In 2013, Gloy et al. reviewed 11 studies comparing surgical and medical treatment of obesity in just under 800 people. The results dramatically favour surgery. On average patients lost 26 kg more weight, and had higher remission rates of diabetes and the metabolic syndrome, greater improvements in quality of life and greater reduction in number of tablets taken. There was also more improvement in cholesterol and triglyceride levels with surgery. Blood pressure did not change significantly.

So you see, surgery is very effective for failures of non-surgical treatment such as repetitive dieting, and I guarantee virtually every one of the surgical patients has been on numerous diets before the surgery. We know however that repetitive dieting is a recipe for one thing, failure. Surgery follows failure. You are going via a different route altogether and if I have anything to do with your outcome you will not be subjected to the surgeon's knife!

# CHAPTER 9

## The Success stories, personal accounts of how and why some people succeed

T HE REASONS SOME people succeed and some people fail when it comes to long term weight loss are numerous and complex. There is a key word here that I am sure you all agree is essential, and this is *motivation.* Without motivation to succeed you are destined to fail. The problem is that everyone seems to be motivated by different things. These may be as far apart as fear of dying in one person, to vanity in another. Stop and think: what it is that is motivating you in the pursuit of weight loss and how might we be able to use this to your advantage?

Remember the old saying I've already used, and repeat it to yourself regularly: "In life there are two types of people, spectators and players". I don't need to remind you, the spectators are the ones sitting watching the TV sport and cheering. The players are out exercising and taking responsibility for their actions, including the type and amount of food they place in their mouth. Which one are you? Which one do you want to be?

You can be passive or active here in response to the problem at hand and what you are prepared to do about it. Did I hear you say, "What problem?" Please put the book down and pick up the TV control; you are wasting your time reading this. If you keep reading the book then by definition you have at least one foot in the "active" camp, we just have to get you to step in with both feet and stay there.

What we need to work out to help you in this is what buttons do we or you need to push to turn on your desire and motivation to achieve weight loss, for good. I will give you a few examples of general principles and some real life case studies of what buttons actually worked in others who are just like you and have success-fully achieved their aim of sustained weight loss. Do any of the case studies sound familiar to you?

*Successful weight loss is said to be associated with:*

- more initial weight loss

- reaching your self-determined goal

- having a physically active life style

- regular meal rhythm including eating breakfast

- healthier eating

- self monitoring behaviours including control of overeating

*Maintenance of weight loss is associated with:*

- internal motivation to lose weight

- social support

- better coping strategies and ability to handle life stress

- assuming personal responsibility for the outcome in life

- overall more psychological strength and stability

- continuing to exercise

*Risk of weight regain is associated with:*

- history of weight cycling (previous failure)

- binge eating

- dietary disinhibition, defined as the tendency to overeat in the presence of palatable foods (conversely, dietary restraint is the tendency to consciously restrict or control food intake)

- eating in response to negative emotions and stress

- a passive approach to dealing with problems.

*Who succeeds in maintaining weight loss? A conceptual review of factors associated with weight loss maintenance and weight regain obesity reviews, 2005 Vol. 6, issue 1*

Clearly, you cannot change all these factors, including your personality. However, you can change some of them or prepare strategies for dealing with them. Look for social support by involving your friends, family or spouse in the program you are undertaking. If you find that you tend to eat when you get negative emotions, then plan to go for a walk instead of eating whenever this occurs and discuss it with those around you and encourage them to help you to enforce your plans. Go through this list and plan how you are going to deal with your own potential liabilities or weaknesses before you take the plunge and make your lifestyle change. A psychologist or lifestyle counsellor may be able to help but it will be primarily up to you. Hopefully you will be more likely to achieve your goal if you plan to succeed, not to fail. Attitude, as I have said and will continue to do so, is very important. The above list is by no means complete and you may be able to add some extra issues you feel may apply to you. The following cases are real life examples of how some people succeeded and what they felt was important in their journey.

## Real life stories

### Control of your own destiny.

Pietro grew up in Australia, the son of two hard working Sicilian migrants in a typical working class environment. His parents had grown up during the Second World War in Europe, often with not enough to eat and were very happy having moved to Australia, "a land of plenty". As migrant families often are, they were a bit isolated, with their mother at home barely able to speak English and their father out working long hours to support them. Their mother was determined that her two sons were not going to have to go through the hardships that she and her husband did. As an expressive Italian mother, her affection for her sons was partly expressed in serving them food: the more they would eat the better, as far as she was concerned. The two sons felt it was their duty to their mother to show their appreciation by eating what they were served. They were after all just doing what was expected of them – nothing more nothing less. It was not really up to them to decide how much to eat, was it?

So Pietro went through his childhood, adolescence and early adulthood doing what was expected. As a result he had a problem with obesity, and as a result of this and his ethnic background life at school was probably not as easy as it might have been. Pietro is a bright fellow and from his humble beginnings went on to study medicine at university. While at university with his medical student colleagues the penny suddenly dropped. He realised all of a sudden that it was actually he who was in control of his own destiny, not his cultural background or any debt to his mother. He was also strong willed and decided one day that enough was enough, he was going to lose weight. He changed his whole outlook on life and eating habits and lost 35-40 kg relatively quickly. That was more than 20 years ago and he has not put one gram back on. His weight has been quite stable in the normal BMI range ever since. All it took was the realisation that he was the one in control of his own destiny; he didn't need anyone else's help or advice.

**Reality shock.**

Sandra is a woman in her mid-50s. She has been overweight most of her adult life and more recently has developed diabetes, high blood pressure and high cholesterol and been put on multiple different tablets, which she dutifully takes. She has been told by her GP and her gastroenterologist (me) that she has to do something about her weight because it will help treat all her other conditions and she will feel much better for it. She does very little exercise, says she eats "almost nothing" and "Yes doctor, I'm doing my best" (this is a recording). She and I had been saying the same thing to one another for at least 10 years, and nothing seemed to change. During this time her weight has gradually increased. Her husband is a truck driver, is the same age and has similar problems. They have three adult children and are happily married.

Then, suddenly, something terrible happened. Her husband, out of the blue, dropped dead from a heart attack. The poor woman was clearly grief stricken but came to terms with what had happened and moved on. Over the next year she lost 40 kg in weight and, like Pietro stabilised her weight in the normal range. That was more than three years ago and she has not regained the weight. She was able to stop all her medications. I have not pushed her for an explanation and have simply been supportive and compassionate. I am not sure exactly what went through her head to lead her to lose weight so quickly and effectively and to keep it off. I sincerely hope you do not need something as drastic to motivate you.

## Body image.

Another patient simply had a picture taken of himself with his daughter, his son in law and son in law's father, at her wedding. He was very shocked when he looked at the picture of himself compared to his son in law's father, who was slim. "Surely that couldn't be me?" This caused him to change his whole outlook on what he had convinced himself was "normal" to such an extent that he too went on to lose a large amount of weight in the next 6 months and has kept if off over the years ever since. The shock changed his body image: he had not even accepted he had a problem up until he looked at the photo.

## I'll show him.

I saw one patient in his mid-40s recently for a minor procedure. I spoke to him for about 5 minutes before the procedure as I usually do but did not recognise him. He reminded me that I had seen him a year ago for a similar procedure and I apologised for not remembering him. He said it was okay, he had been 47 kg heavier a year ago. Amazed, I immediately inquired as to how and what he had done to achieve this, as always hoping to learn something. He replied, "Some rude bastard told me I was too fat a year ago". No prizes for guessing who that rude bastard was. Unfortunately he would not tell me what I had said so I could use the same line on others. I cannot remember the discussion.

### Relationship issues.

Chris is a friend of one of my sons, aged 19. He had a significant weight problem and had finally decided to do something about it, prompted by relationship problems and his feelings of rejection. He is a strong willed fellow. He looked at what he was doing wrong and decided to reduce his portion size and began aerobic and weight training exercises. Within 8 months he had lost 75 kg. He feels the portion size reduction was the greatest benefit. This was more than 12 months ago and he has not put a gram back on, he just continues with his change in lifestyle. He continues to smile!

### Am I really hungry?

Robin is a doctor who I work with. She gives anaesthetics for my medical procedures. With a medical background she was well aware of the pitfalls of obesity. When she had moved to Japan as a younger woman she found the food delicious. Before she really realised what was happening she had put on 30 kg in weight and after several years decided she had to do something about the issue. From then on every time she went to eat she asked herself,

"Am I really hungry?" If not, she didn't eat. Within 12 months she had lost all the excess weight and more. That was about 30 years ago and she has put none of the weight back on again. This is an important concept I will touch on again later in the book.

These are just a few stories from my friends and family, you will know of others who have similar stories. If it wasn't possible to lose weight these stories would not be so common. Have a think about them. What is your trigger or switch? How do we turn it on?

# CHAPTER 10

## How to put it all together. The recipe for sustained weight loss and the rules to follow

NONE OF THIS chapter should surprise you and I am sure many of you will say, "I've heard it all before! Why is this any different?" Well, I am hoping that the difference this time is that you are not going to just be "hearing" it; you are going to be "doing" it. As a doctor having spent 30 years discussing issues with patients it never ceases to amaze me how often the patients seem to think these are the same thing. They just go to their doctor to be told what they have to do, they never do it. Well, I am sure you know there is a difference. That difference is the difference between success and failure. Now not only do we want you to do these things, we want you to do them forever – that is, if you are lucky enough to live that long.

This is what I would call "lifestyle change". It is not a short term diet. However, what you put in your mouth is by far the most important part of sustained weight loss.

## 1. Don't eat processed food.

This is the most important message in the book and I don't apologise for repeating it over and over.

How do you recognise processed foods? Well that is not really very difficult is it? Processed foods are the ones in packets, in cans or in bottles or other packaging. Some things in packets are obviously fine, such as the freshly frozen vegetables. However, read the packet to make sure that it is all there is in the packet. Tinned tomatoes sound safe enough, but make sure that is all they are and take the ones with no added sugar or salt! Learn to read labels carefully and critically.

Keep in your mind what the food giants do to get you to eat these foods and why they taste so good. Remember, they have done lots of research, on both rats and people, to sort out what you find irresistible so that you eat as much as possible and keep coming back for more, just like the rats. With these foods you are not likely to be able to restrict your portion size effectively, with obvious results. So please do not put yourself in that position. Do you want to win or lose this fight? The combinations they have come up with are the ones not found in nature so evolution gave you no effective off switch, you just keep eating until you cannot physically fit any more in your stomach. They are usually combinations of fat and sugar in that magic proportion of about half and half and the combination of fat and salt. They also use many chemical flavour enhancers such as monosodium glutamate or msg. With a name like that it couldn't possibly be good for you, could it? Why do you think those fried potato chips or donuts taste so good? Just one more ...

If you want to eat processed food, then process it yourself. At least that way you'll know, and have some control, over what is in it. If you have to learn to cook, then so be it. If you have to make time to cook, then make time. Haven't we already used the phrase, "You are a long time dead"? One thing is almost certain: you are likely to be dead sooner if you eat processed foods. Then it may be a bit hard to learn to cook, even if you do have the time! If you are going to buy processed food then do it as infrequently as possible, feel as guilty as possible and READ the ingredients before you buy it. Remind yourself what things like trans-fatty acids are and what they can do to you. Hopefully this will shock you so badly you will put it back on the shelf for some other poor, less aware sucker to buy. He or she can then keep the heart doctors and undertakers busy. I'm sure you would rather not be their clients yourself.

Processed food means any food that has been adulterated, be it the "reduced fat" (heavily sugared) yogurt or the "toasted" (high fat) muesli described earlier, the hamburgers or the pizzas. Go back to basics and buy fresh or freshly frozen vegetables, fish, meat or chicken and use your imagination. Make your own muesli. Sticking a hole in a bag of frozen mixed vegetables and then putting them in the microwave for 5 minutes is not very difficult, while you steam or fry with minimum oil (spray on) your fish, chicken or meat. The fresh frozen vegetables are just as good for you as the fresh ones from the supermarket, and they are easier to keep. You might even add some herbs or spices. Use your imagination. I can cook a meal in less than 10 minutes, much quicker than driving for takeaway, and I am sure you can too.

## 2. Eat upside down.

Well, not really: what I want is for you to turn your eating habits upside down.

### a) Daily eating habits

This is a very important concept that I think is crucial for sustained weight loss and the evidence is now mounting to support it. It is not yet in the general media as far as I am aware. Let me walk you through it. You do not have to conform to society's norms in your eating behaviour.

Most of us have three meals per day and you would think that if we simply dropped one of these we would lose weight, and you are right. But it is very important which one we drop. Many people skip breakfast, for all sorts of reasons including time, lack of hunger, weight loss or just habit. This should make them thinner, shouldn't it? Well, unfortunately the reverse is true. People who skip breakfast seem to end up more obese than people who eat it regularly. The majority of research studies, but not all, show this. Not really fair, is it? The other unfortunate thing is that the effect seems to be greater in children and adolescents than in older adults, setting the young up for obesity in later life. In one study of over 35,000 Dutch adolescents, the risk of being overweight was 2.17 times greater if the adolescents skipped breakfast. In other words, they were twice as likely to be overweight if they skipped breakfast.

*S. Croezen, European Journal of Clinical Nutrition 2009.*

The second problem with skipping breakfast, especially in children, is that things in your body that run on glucose don't function as well. Yes, I am talking about your brain. Numerous studies show that children do not do as well at school in exams and other tests of brain function if they do not eat breakfast. I'm sure the same is true for adults and, if you are anything like me, we need all the help we can get, especially in the morning!

So it is settled: you cannot go skipping breakfast. In fact you can probably have as large a breakfast as you like.

So if you cannot skip breakfast, what about lunch? Well, the evidence is mixed here. Those against will argue that if you miss lunch you put yourself in starvation mode and reduce your metabolic rate, and this is associated with a marked increase in appetite. The result in many studies is that you tend to overeat snacks during the afternoon and, worse still, when you are hungry you will go for the unhealthy high energy choices such as biscuits, which are really just flour, fat and sugar, possibly making you worse off in the long run. The other concern is that you will be so hungry when you get home that you have a very large evening meal to make up and this has potentially alarming metabolic consequences such as increasing your risk of developing diabetes.

There are studies published showing that skipping lunch is effective for weight loss. However, you have to be disciplined because of the increased hunger, which will ease with time as this becomes a habit. If you stick to a normal sized evening meal you will reduce you energy intake by 30% and you will lose weight. Interestingly, it also seems to improve your asthma. None of these studies looked at cheating with things like inulin and cocoa as I have described to make it easier.

*Free Radical Biology and Medicine, 2007.*

The other advantages of skipping lunch include the fact that it is by far the easiest meal to skip as most people are at work. You might like to think your body goes into "starvation mode", but this in reality takes at least 24 hours or more. It is also a great time to get out and exercise. Go for a long walk or a run, walk up and down the stairs of the office, go shopping for your smaller clothes (not food). You will still feel hungry but the activities described will distract you somewhat and feeling hungry is not the end of the world, you will get used to it. If you want to take something to supress your hunger then take a fibre supplement like chicory root extract, one rounded dessert spoon with a rounded dessert spoon of cocoa, mixed in water or skim milk, hot or cold an hour before you were due to eat. This works. I have tried it. I only skipped lunch for a week to see how easy it was and took my belt in two holes, but I confess I did not weigh myself. I found the cocoa very effective at supressing hunger. However, if you take too much you will feel nauseated. The stimulant effect of the cocoa meant I was much more awake and energised than if I had eaten! I didn't eat at all in the afternoons and did not have a larger evening meal. In fact, I often felt less hungry than if I had had lunch. I felt I could easily continue this indefinitely. If however you are going to end up by having a much larger evening meal then you may do yourself much more harm than good because of increased risk of developing many features of the metabolic syndrome.

In summary, skipping lunch is a viable weight loss strategy but only if you are going to be disciplined in what you do for the rest of the day. It is not that hard.

So this brings us to the obvious conclusion that if breakfast is definitely out, lunch is a possibility, what about the evening meal? Well, I think this has huge potential for effective weight loss. The problem is this is often a social occasion with friends and family, making it much harder to miss than lunch. If you can do it with appetite suppressants like cocoa and bulking agents like inulin or Konjac then you are well on the way to success and this is likely to be highly effective. You do not need those calories to sleep and you will likely sleep more peacefully. It is also hard to eat in your sleep, but I would padlock the fridge and cupboards just in case you mysteriously develop sleep walking habits!

An alternative half way house is to do as suggested and turn eating habits upside down. What I mean here is a large breakfast, smaller lunch and even smaller dinner, NOT the other way around as most of us do now. Your evening meal should be a very small piece of fish, chicken or meat and some low calorie vegetables, such as bok choy, onions, celery, broccoli, which you can throw in the pan and fry with the fish, having sprayed a tiny bit of oil in the non-stick pan. If this is simply not enough then put a packet of Konjac noodles in the pan as well. These are only 0.8 calories per gram so you can fill up on them and they taste just like rice noodles. This is only a suggestion: you are allowed to use your imagination. That is it: no snacking later. Take the appetite suppressants or bulking agents if you must. Go for a walk.

I can only find one article at present to justify this approach but I think it is likely that more will follow. Jakubowicz and colleagues published in the journal *Obesity* in March of 2013. They took 93 overweight or obese women with the metabolic syndrome and randomised them to two different meal plans, both with the same number of calories and food content, one with most of the food for breakfast and the other with most of the food for dinner. They were followed for 12 weeks and this was a "diet", but I think the results can be extrapolated long term. Both groups had 1400 Kcal, split 700/500/200 for breakfast/lunch/dinner for the breakfast group and the reverse for the dinner group. The results were impressive. The breakfast group lost twice as much weight as the dinner group with a 10% drop in BMI in the breakfast group compared to a 5% drop in the dinner group. The breakfast group also had greater loss of waist circumference, lower blood sugar and much lower blood fats or triglycerides, the latter actually increasing in the dinner group. There was greater improvement in almost all features of the metabolic syndrome in the breakfast group. Not only this, but do you know which group had much less hunger during the diet? That's right: the breakfast group found the diet much easier to follow and scored significantly higher on satiety scores.

So you see, we have it all wrong. We should be having a large breakfast, small lunch and even smaller dinner, if we have the dinner at all.

### b)  Weekly eating habits
#### Intermittent fasting-calorie restriction

No discussion on changing your eating habits is complete without addressing this issue which has been gaining popularity recently. This is at least as effective as daily calorie restriction, if not more so, for weight loss and control of all the parameters of the metabolic syndrome. There are no long term (years) studies I am aware of. The positive effects are well documented in animal and human studies.

On the positive side is the fact that during the days you are not restricting calories you can eat what you like – but I would still strongly advise: try to stick to most of the calories early in the day if possible - and remember, you should really not be exceeding 2500 calories for males and 2000 for females on these "free" days.

One possible negative is that you are doing different things on different days, in other words not getting into a fixed daily lifestyle or routine, with concerns about long term compliance. Having said this the diet certainly seems to be well adhered to and effective in the short term – months.

There are a number of ways of doing this. Initially it was tried as an alternative day regime however a 5:2 approach is now more popular. This means that for 2 days per week, not necessarily consecutive, you restrict yourself to less than 600 calories for males or less than 500 calories for females. You would still be allowed to take your inulin and cocoa but remember the inulin is about 1 calorie per gram.

So what do you eat on the calorie restricted days? Well I would focus on protein and fat not carbohydrate. For breakfast you might have a small tin of salmon or tuna (100g is about 150 calories – in water or brine not oil), half an avocado for lunch (120-150 calories) and a hand full of nuts for the evening meal (150 calories). Things like lettuce salads, spinach leaves have very few calories and could be combined with the other suggestions above, but that's it for those 2 days. Don't forget there are calories in drinks too so ideally your tea, coffee or cocoa should be black or only a tiny splash of milk. If you do use appetite suppressants like cocoa and bulking agents like inulin to fill you up between meals, perhaps for morning and afternoon breaks, then this will be easier to adhere to.

So if short periods of fasting work, why not just go for longer? Surely more is better? Well you are correct that this would result in more weight loss but you would lose large amounts of muscle bulk as well with your being very likely to rebound in weight. Your body has no choice but to use up your muscles to make glucose, without which you would die. Remember muscle is your friend in this long term battle to lose weight and keep the weight off, it burns calories even while you sleep. Maintaining your so called "lean body mass" is very important, it keeps your metabolic rate or energy burning rate higher. Questions would also arise about long term adherence to this strategy. Short term - one day at a time - seems to be the best of both worlds. It preserves muscle bulk and works for weight loss and the metabolic syndrome, including your diabetes.

If you can stick to an intermittent fasting/calorie restriction regime you will lose weight so why don't you give it a go, perhaps every Tuesday and Thursday starting next week. If you do this when you are distracted at work it will be much easier to adhere to than weekends or holidays where temptations undoubtedly will arise. If you don't think you can stick to this type of program long term then don't try, we are only interested in long term results and permanent changes to your lifestyle. The authors of the reference below give quite a good review of this topic and the evidence for its use. Read it if you are interested in more detail than I have given here.

*The British Journal of Diabetes & Vascular Disease 2013(2), 68-72*

THE MYSTERY OF SUSTAINED WEIGHT LOSS...

## 3. Don't allow processed food or junk food in the house.

When you sit down at the end of a hard day to have a chat to your partner or watch the TV and relax you are often at your weakest. As far as you are concerned there are other much more important things on your mind than what you put in your mouth. If you don't have any biscuits, sweets, cakes, chocolate, chips, soft drink or processed foods of other sorts at home it makes it much harder for you to eat them. If you do have healthy alternatives you'll just have to make do with those instead, as per some of the suggestions in food substitutions.

How successful do you think you are going to be at restricting you calories in the evening if you fill the house with junk?!

You must plan ahead if you are going to be successful. When you walk into the house after a day's work it is too late. For goodness sakes, plan to succeed not to fail, and don't fail to plan.

## 4. Dessert is for special occasions only.

Who said you had to have a three course meal in the evenings? Having dessert or sweets or pudding after your evening meal is far from a necessity and should be considered a luxury only for special occasions such as birthdays or other celebrations. If you want something after your evening meal then try some fruit (in moderation) or some low calorie alternative such as carrot and celery sticks or even one of the bulking agents previously described to fill you up. You will get over missing dessert and it will be normal for you not to have it. If you are going to have this try to do it away from home. One ice cream in a cone is not as bad as having a whole bucket in the freezer. If you put it in the freezer it won't stay there for long!

## 5. Don't drink fruit juice or allow it in the house.

There is a reason for fructose and fruit beginning the same way. Fructose gets its name from the same derivation as fruit (from the Latin fructus) and really stands for "fruit sugar". This is where nearly all the calories in the fruit lie. The drink in the supermarket with the most sugar is not the soft drink or soda, it is the processed, mixed and often sweetened long life fruit juices. There is nearly a whole aisle of these. The kids love them because they are sweet and the parents of the kids think they are doing their children or themselves a favour with "natural" fruit juice. Well I am afraid they are sadly mistaken. Their makers want you to think they are healthy. That way you will buy them. The fact is they are very bad. Remember what happens when you consume a large amount of fructose? Where does it go?

If you want to think of this another way, one apple is good for you because the fructose is slowly absorbed from the solid apple pieces and dealt with. Do you think 20 apples are good for you? How quickly can you drink a litre of cold apple juice when you are really thirsty? Not that hard, is it? The calories from 20 apples down the hatch in a jiffy. Not just any calories, but almost all fructose, really bad stuff, and to make matters worse it is absorbed almost immediately as it is dissolved in water. Your body has no option except to turn it straight into fat in your liver and abdomen. Now try eating 20 apples. Not that easy, is it? Fruit was meant for eating, NOT DRINKING. Just because it is "natural" does not mean it is good for you in large amounts. Arsenic and cyanide are "natural" too. They are not very good for you in large amounts either. Fruit juice is another processed food and it is no better for you if you juice it at home, so just stick to the low calorie vegetables like celery when using your juicer (or better still throw the juicer out).

## 6. Don't eat unless you are hungry. EVERY time you eat, ask yourself, "Am I really hungry?"

This seems simple, but nothing is ever as simple as it seems. People eat for all sorts of reasons: out of habit; when they are nervous; for social reasons; as comfort food and many others. You must be aware of this and think of it EVERY time you put something in your mouth. "Am I really hungry?"

If you are not hungry, don't eat. If you are full, stop eating. You do not have to eat everything on your plate just because it was put in front of you or your mother told you to 20 years ago. Remember, you are the one in control of your own destiny. If you do feel like eating then make up a simple rule to use like the "apple rule" and live by it. If you are not hungry enough to eat an apple then you are not really hungry. If you are hungry enough to eat the apple then eat the apple, not the potato chips! Alternatively, you could try a fibre drink like inulin one dessert spoon in a glass of water, but add a teaspoon or two of cocoa as an appetite suppressant. This will take about an hour to work, but when the inulin gets to your colon in 6 hours it also supresses your appetite further.

Missing meals can be a very effective weight loss strategy but I would suggest an appetite suppressant such as cocoa powder and, as discussed above, missing breakfast seems to be too hard for most people. You must be disciplined. Lunch is a very real alternative, especially if you are working. Dinner is even better but harder to do socially.

You may be surprised to learn that if you drink only water and eat nothing it takes about 6 weeks (not 6 minutes) before any potentially serious medical issues arise, and that is for people with a BMI in the normal range. So stop feeling sorry for yourself! Remember being slightly hungry is not the end of the world, you'll get used to it.

## 7. Get enough sleep.

Sleep and obesity are complex issues that are likely to be inversely related. The science is still evolving but there seems to be little doubt that lack of sleep or poor sleep quality are very real risk factors for developing obesity. Generally, the larger people are, the less quality sleep they get. This is because of a condition called sleep apnoea, where the airway becomes obstructed when they are asleep and they need to keep waking up to breathe. This is strongly correlated with obesity and the metabolic syndrome. We now believe that 7 hours of sleep, not 8, is the optimal amount. Any less and you impair cognitive performance and memory, as well as increasing your risk of obesity. Any more than 7 hours of sleep and you can show increased risk of obesity, diabetes, cardiovascular disease and death. The problem here, some will argue, is one of the "chicken and egg" phenomena. Sick people are more at risk of dying and likely to need more sleep: would seem obvious, wouldn't it? Some would say we are confusing causation and association here. It is probably a real finding, however. Prospective studies, that are likely to be correct, going for over 10 years, show that if you get less than 5 hours of sleep or more than 6.5 hours of sleep you are more likely to die.

---

*2011 Kripke et al., Sleep medicine.*

When it comes to obesity the bottom of the graph for weight, when weight is graphed against sleep duration, is about 6.5-7 hours. It is a U shaped curve. The effect of increasing weight on moving either side of this point is more pronounced for going down in hours' sleep than up.

The obesity epidemic has occurred at a time when people in our society are getting less sleep and less quality sleep. In studies looking at what happens if you take human volunteers and restrict sleep, they have changes in hormones that control appetite such as leptin and ghrelin, their appetite and hunger levels increase and they will eat more. You can show the same in animal studies with rats. Not only do the people and the rats eat more when sleep deprived but they seem to go for the unhealthy, carbohydrate rich foods.

Remember, we are discussing volunteers here with normal BMI, not larger people with sleep apnoea. Once you add sleep apnoea to the picture it may become self-perpetuating. That is to say, the larger you get, the worse the sleep apnoea, resulting in less quality sleep. The less quality sleep you get the stronger your appetite or hunger levels get, resulting in excessive food intake. This is a bit like the brakes failing in your car while driving down a hill: you go faster and faster and faster down the hill, out of control. You can interchange the unit kilometres per hour (KPH) for BMI. Your choice, they both keep rising. I hope you are not going to hit anything too hard when you get to the bottom of that hill.

Sleep deficit not only makes you gain weight, it increases your likelihood of developing diabetes and other elements of the metabolic syndrome. This may relate to increases in the levels of the hormone cortisol, the body's stress hormone, which occurs with sleep deprivation. All the above effects seem to be more pronounced in children and young adults, setting them up for more diseases later in life.

So how much sleep do you need? Well 7 hours is probably the magic amount. Once you get less than 6 hours it is easy to show effects, including increased appetite and the risk of obesity.

Unfortunately for you there is no evidence that getting more than 7 hours sleep aids in weight loss and, in fact, as described, the reverse is true, where too much sleep may be harmful.

If you want to read some of the evidence for these claims there are hundreds of studies on sleep research in the medical research literature. One example is a meta-analysis or pooled results from 18 similar studies involving more than 600,000 adults. This showed a 1.55 times increased risk of obesity with less than 5 hours sleep per night and also a progressive inverse effect, where the less sleep you had the higher the BMI is likely to be.

*Cappuccio, Oxford University Press, Oxford, pp. 83-110.*

Now believe it or not, I am not dwelling on this to put you to sleep. To summarise the literature, you should aim for at least 6, preferably 7 hours of quality sleep per night. Any less and you increase levels of the stress hormone cortisol, contributing to increased risk of diabetes (decreased insulin sensitivity), increased levels of the hunger hormone ghrelin and decreased levels of the hunger supressing hormone leptin with resultant increase in appetite, hunger and weight.

Short sleep duration is particularly associated with increased risk of obesity. Please turn off the TV or put your book down and go to bed!

## 8. *Don't take antibiotic medication unless you really need it.*

Now this comment is not evidence based but I think will be proven to be correct, at least in theory, in the longer term. It applies perhaps more to your children than to you. Having said this, you should always do as your doctor advises. Taking antibiotics for a viral infection such as a common cold however is not helpful and may be harmful. Doctors have a tendency to do what patients want them to do so if you go asking for antibiotics as the cold has "gone to my chest" you are likely to be given them by some doctors to get you out the door. Explanations take a long time, especially when the patient has already decided the opposite to what you are trying to explain and you are an hour behind with a full waiting room.

The point here is the faecal microbiome, or if you like all the bugs living inside you in your gut. Remember, they outnumber the number of cells in your body many times over. The number of different species of bacteria, or the diversity present in the gut of an obese person, is very different from a thin person. The difference is in both type of bugs and the number of bugs. However, generally speaking, the fatter you are the fewer species of bacteria you have living in your bowel. The difference is very impressive, often by a factor of 10 or 50 times. When you look at African natives living traditional lifestyles and compare them to Northern Americans living in large clean cities with flushing toilets, then there is a very large difference between the type and number of

bacteria living in the bowel, with the traditional Africans having far more. The difference is not just between individuals, it
is between societies. We are not only speaking about the difference between fat and thin individuals, we are also able to draw
comparisons between fat and thin societies. The same applies:
the larger the people in a society the fewer species of bacteria in
their bowel. North Americans have far less diverse types of bugs
in the bowel compared to traditional African natives.

So if obese people and obese societies have far fewer types of bacteria in the bowel, could this be partly responsible for the obesity epidemic? The answer is probably yes, as has already been
discussed in the text of this book. Remember, some bacteria produce products such as short chain fatty acids that cause a release
of hormone peptides from the lining of the gut, such as GLP1,
which have an effect on appetite or hunger by acting directly on
the brain's appetite centre.

No prize for guessing who is most likely to have this type of
bacteria in the bowel: the thin or the obese individual, the thin
or obese society?

So what is the most effective way to kill bacteria, good and bad?
Would that be antibiotics? The evidence is mounting that overuse of antibiotics in society may be causally related to the obesity
epidemic. There are many who believe that a risk factor for obesity, if not the cause of the epidemic, is the overuse of antibiotics
in children, with the number of courses of antibiotics correlating
with the longer term risk of obesity.

The same is probably true of animals. Chicken farmers have known for years that if you mix antibiotics such as vancomycin in the chicken feed the chickens grow and fatten up very much more quickly than if you do not use antibiotics. The result is fat succulent chickens grown in half the time, and the serious issue of antibiotic resistant bacteria that we cannot treat when these resistant bacteria infect humans. The same is true of cattle and pigs fed in feed lots. As with everything else it is all about money and profits, to hell with the consequences, not the point of this book but a reason to push for legislation to ban such practices. The battery and feed lot owners pretend it "stops them from getting sick" but they are not sick to start with. It probably works by altering the bacteria in the bowel and inducing a strong appetite and altering the animal's metabolism. We know that changing the bacteria in the bowel can do this.

So the next obvious question is, "Can I get the cocktail of bugs to make me thin, and if so how?" Well the answer may well be yes in the very near future, but you may be a bit shocked to know how we would do this, so I will leave it out for now. Altering the bowel's bacteria in animal studies works, inducing weight loss or weight gain as above. Remember it has not been proven in humans that this is an effective way to treat obesity. This is partly because it has not been done! Watch this space: the potential for an effective treatment is real. Until then try to look after the bugs in your bowel. They are much more important than you think, not only for the potential of weight control but many other functions as well.

## 9. Shopping rules

### a) *Never shop when you are hungry.*

There are many studies looking at this issue. The bottom line is that if you go shopping when you are hungry you are more likely to buy higher calorie, less healthy foods, so why make it hard for yourself. This is about the only point in the book where I will actually tell you to have a healthy snack, so do so BEFORE you go shopping. Again, you could use cocoa one hour before you shop.

This has been looked at with hungry and fed volunteers in real and virtual supermarkets. It has even been shown that the time of day you go shopping changes your choices: the later in the afternoon you shop (presumably when you are further from your lunch), the less healthy and higher calorie choices you are likely to make.

---

*JAMA May 2013 online*

### b) *Always shop from a list, NO browsing!*

Before you go shopping you should think about what you really need and write a list. Plan your meals ahead of time. If you go wandering aimlessly down the supermarket aisles you are likely to fall prey to the supermarket advertising. This advertising is carefully planned and placed to take you in. It is tried and proven to work. It will take you in. You are not as clever as you think! So watch out for unhealthy food which is "on special today only half price ...". You don't need it, so don't buy it! Just buy the things on your list.

### c) Shop around the edges of the supermarket aisles.

If you walk around the edge of the supermarket you are likely to encounter the dairy products, meats and seafood, breads, fresh fruits and vegetables. You should only go down the aisles to get the extras on your list like the cocoa. Why shouldn't you go down the aisles? You haven't been listening, have you? The aisles are where all the processed food is! Stay away from the advertising. Stay away from the processed foods!

## 10. Eating rules

### a) Use smaller plates and bowls.

Give the others away to someone who is anorexic or throw them out so you cannot access them again. This is not simply a matter of not being physically able to put any more on your plate. It is actually quite clever psychology. If you put the same amount of food on a smaller plate it actually looks like more food and you are more likely to be satisfied. Conversely, if you pick up a larger plate and use this you will fill it until it looks about right to you, which is significantly more food.

Research has shown that generally people eat about 92% of what they place on their plates, regardless of the size of the plate. If you reduce the size of the plate from 30 cm (12 inches) to 25 cm (10 inches) people have been shown to serve themselves 22% less food. Over 12 months this alone would result in weight loss of 8.4 kg or 18 lbs. It is not enough of a reduction to trigger a hunger response, especially as you tend to be fooled because the plate looks much fuller and you think you are getting about the same.

———————

*JAMA April 2005*

Control of portion size has been shown in numerous studies to be an effective weight loss strategy. Smaller plates and bowls is just one suggestion of how to make it easier for you to reduce your portion size. You may have others. Stop and think about how to achieve this.

### b)  *Eat a small amount of protein with every meal.*

Protein is something you cannot put away for a rainy day: you either use it to maintain your muscle mass, or you break it down and burn it for energy. On the other hand, fat and carbohydrate you can store away, especially the fat, where the storage capacity is virtually limitless. Protein is one of the most effective food types to cause satiety or a feeling of fullness, which results in you stopping eating and keeps you feeling satisfied for longer, potentially avoiding unnecessary snacks before the next meal. Just to prove this to yourself, have a piece of fish, chicken or meat and wait for the signal from your body telling you to stop eating. Then for another meal sit down in front of a large plate of fried potato chips with salt. There was virtually no protein in the second meal and I'll bet you got no off signal until you had finished the plate and then you went looking for more. As a result you got about five times as many calories for your trouble! Grasshoppers are just the same. They eat continuously until they get a sufficient amount of protein and then stop eating, even if it means taking in 3 times as much carbohydrate to get it!

The second thing that happens if you eat small amounts of protein regularly is that you inhibit loss of your muscle bulk. Carbohydrate does the same, but you only need very small amounts of this, taken as complex carbohydrate not sugar. So use protein, as it works better and you won't take in too many carbs. Remember, your muscles are very useful in aiding your quest for weight loss, particularly of fat. They keep burning energy even while you are sleeping, just to keep themselves alive. Now you do not have to eat large amounts of protein for this effect, nor do I want you to because large amounts may be harmful over the longer term. A small glass of skim milk for example would be more than adequate with your meal if the rest of the meal contains no protein.

### c) Eat slowly. Put down the fork and talk!

As discussed above, you have built in mechanisms to assess when you have had enough to eat, which involve all the major food groups but, as discussed, protein is the most effective one of these. The problem is these take time, probably about 45 minutes, to cut in and in a busy lifestyle this is a lot of time. By then most people have just kept eating until they feel full because they have started to physically run out of room for more food in their stomach. If they had waited longer they would have felt full and been able to push the plate away without emptying it, because of chemical messengers coming back from the brain and elsewhere saying: "Enough is enough!"

### d) Stop eating 3 hours before going to bed.

This is assuming you have to eat at all in the evening. Eating immediately before going to bed is not a healthy thing to do. To begin with, when you lie flat with a full stomach it is likely some of this is going to reflux into your oesophagus or swallowing tube. This reflux, apart from causing many people troublesome symptoms, increases your risk of developing oesophageal cancer.

The food being absorbed while you are asleep doesn't have many options for use. It goes into storage for later use, as you don't really need it at the time. You would be much better off eating early and going for a walk. You will sleep better with the exercise, and you may also sleep better because some of the chemicals in the food may interfere with you sleeping and keep you awake. You try it: I'll bet you sleep well if you don't eat immediately before retiring. Remember, the quality of your sleep is very important if you are to succeed in your aim of weight loss long term. There are many potential benefits to eating earlier, if this is possible for you in your busy lifestyle.

## 11. Get in the zone, repetitively remind yourself of your goal.

You cannot take your eye off the ball if you are playing this game for keeps. You need to keep reinforcing what your aim is and why. You need to learn to think thin and change your whole perception of what you now think is "normal" for you. The people who take a keen interest in this process are the ones who succeed. They are likely to alter their brain structure permanently. Then it just feels normal. To help reinforce this brain change you should do the following.

*a)* *Weigh yourself every week and write it down in your journal with the date.*

Make it the same time, perhaps when you have a shower in the mornings.

b) *Calorie count and keep a food journal of everything you eat every day.*

You may be very surprised when you look back at how well you are really following these rules and hopefully the associated guilt will make you reconsider your behaviour. You might think you are following the instructions to the letter. If you do monitor your progress critically and honestly, you are much more likely to follow the rules and consequently to be successful.

Those people who carefully and obsessively follow their progress and calorie count are much more likely to be successful in weight loss long term. Many studies show this. I have given you all the information you need to do this in terms of how energy dense carbohydrate, fat and protein are in earlier chapters. When I use the term calories, strictly speaking these are termed kilocalories. The conversion between Kilocalories and Kilojoules is 4.18, if the figures on the food packet you are looking at are in Kilojoules. Generally speaking the figures on the packet will be documented per 100g so all you need is a set of accurate kitchen scales to weigh the food and document what you are actually eating.

There are nutritional guidelines about how much energy you should be consuming. These are general guidelines only. They are influenced by your sex, your age, your height, your weight and your level of physical activity. As a very rough guide: women need about 2000 calories per day and men about 2500. The breakdown of the food components in your diet I would advise for normal weight healthy people is about 60% complex carbohydrate (not sugar),

20-30% fat and 10-20% protein. As will be discussed in point 16 if you are diabetic or having trouble losing excess weight you are not in this category, well not yet anyway. Consequently these general "nutritional guidelines" do not apply to you. You need to reduce the carbohydrate component in your diet and increase the protein and fat components, while also reducing your total calorific intake. How severely you do this depends on how difficult your diabetes is to control or how bad the other features of the metabolic syndrome are where you as an individual are concerned.

What I would like you to do is write down what you are doing now, before initiating the 17 point plan, and keep a record after beginning, at least for the first 3 months. This ensures you are taking a detailed interest in what is going on and this will become natural for you in the long run. If you are not losing weight you are doing something wrong and you can take all your records to your doctor or dietician to discuss the issue. They will help you sort this out. If your dietician says, as many patients of mine tell me they do: "you are not eating enough", or "you need to eat more carbohydrate", then get another dietician. They are not on your side. There is no magic here, only simple common sense and simple mathematics.

### c) Talk to others about your aim.

The more you talk about this issue the more you will reinforce it in your brain and the more likely you are to succeed. You don't want to drive all your friends away but hopefully your partner or good friend can support you and offer encouragement.

## 12. *Embark on this quest with another person(s).*

If you do this in a group you can support each other and you can have likeminded discussions about your progress. If you are tempted to pull out or give up you are not just letting yourself down, you are letting the whole group down and this can be a strong motivator, especially if the other person is someone you love or feel strongly about. You must keep in mind that you are doing this for yourself primarily but there is nothing wrong with the whole family being involved, especially if they all have the same problem, as is often the case.

## 13. *Exercise regularly.*

As I have discussed, studies show that exercise alone is not a very effective way of losing weight. As this list would suggest, however, we are not discussing doing "exercise alone". The combination is very helpful, both for your general wellbeing and for your weight. It seems to work better at stopping you regaining the weight you have lost than losing weight. The difficulty with using exercise alone to lose weight is related to compensatory mechanisms that increase your appetite. There are two different types of exercise we need to consider and you should aim to do a mixture of both of these.

Aerobic exercise, such as jogging, swimming, or walking quickly, is very good for you and very good at preventing the diseases associated with obesity such as diabetes. You have to do a large amount of exercise to lose a small amount of weight, but remember you have the rest of your life to do it in and these "small amounts" add up, and up and up. This is probably the reason people who exercise regularly seem to be better at stopping weight regain.

Physical training with weights builds muscle. Muscle bulk is your best friend here. You lose it very quickly if you stop exercising, but while you have it, it will continue to keep your metabolic rate up and help you lose that weight, so don't stop! Remember, that extra muscle is burning extra calories every minute of the day, even when you are asleep.

In terms of direct advice about how much exercise, refer to the chapter on this topic, but this should be part of your daily routine. Yes that is right, if possible EVERY DAY, the more the better, within reason. I would aim for at least 45 minutes per day. Don't have the time? That's okay. Remember again, you will have all the time in the world once you are dead, but it may be a bit harder to do those sit ups. There is also a special reimbursement scheme that has been set up for people just like you. For every 45 minutes exercising you will get to live about 45 minutes longer, so you see, you don't lose any time at all, you get it all back! You are also healthier, so you will be able to make more of that time you are not exercising in your life! Get off your arse and get out there! How much time are you spending on the computer and TV per day?

## 14. Actively practise food substitution.

We have already touched on this but you need to actively think about it every time you go to prepare food or serve food for yourself. This includes making sensible choices: have the leafy spinach and broccoli, not the sweet and floury vegetables such as potato and pumpkin. Don't put your curry on rice, put it on a pile of steamed vegetables instead. The only thing limiting you here is your imagination. If you say you don't have any imagination then google "healthy choices for rice, pasta, potatoes ...". You will be amazed at what turns up. If you like rice and pasta, then look for Konjac noodles in the supermarket and substitute these. It is all out there, you just have to look.

The ultimate food substitution is simply to miss a meal – yes the evening meal – but take the tablespoon of cocoa and inulin at least an hour before the meal and drink plenty of water.

## 15. Alcohol.

I expect you were waiting for this one. There is no question alcohol contains energy. Remember, it is 7 calories per gram, which is not far behind fat. There is no question drinking a lot of alcohol makes you obese, in all the wrong places. I'm sure you have heard of the term "beer belly", although some of this may relate to the sugar in the beer. One option is simply to give it up, and this would certainly help with weight loss. The other is to restrict yourself to 1-2 standard drinks per day, preferably avoiding beer and mixed drinks, which are also loaded with sugar. The reason for my being a bit soft with this suggestion is the evidence that 1-2 drinks per day reduces your risk of dying from vascular disease such as strokes and heart attacks. Any alcohol increases your risk of many cancers; however, as more people die from vascular disease, overall you are less likely to die. Once you go over two standard drinks you are more likely to die from all causes, so 1-2 means 1-2, NOT 2-3 or any larger number you care to mention.

## 16. Spice up your life

Well, at least your food. We have discussed how the capsaicin in chilli may increase your metabolic rate by causing meal-induced thermogenesis and by stimulating brown fat which may increase your basal metabolic rate. Some studies suggest mustard may also do this, more so than chilli. There are studies showing that if you eat chilli in most of your food you tend to feel more satisfied and eat significantly less at subsequent meals. There are numerous claims about other spices in the literature such as tumeric and weight loss and many of these may relate to stimulation of your sense of smell which results in satiety or feeling satisfied with how much you have eaten earlier. This results in fewer calories and potential weight loss. But don't stop at chilli, make sure your pantry has numerous spices and use them liberally as they may well help you feel full and reduce your portion size. These include mustard, garlic, ginger, cardamom, turmeric, black pepper, cayenne pepper, cumin, coriander, lemon grass and many others. You can put in as much as you like, they have minimal if any calories themselves.

## 17. Carbohydrate is the enemy.

As I keep trying to convince you, the "Metabolic Syndrome" could certainly be defined as a "Carbohydrate Poisoning Syndrome" or an "Exercise deficiency state". Take your pick. We are focusing here on the first of these two definitions.

This is not the last point in the list because it is least important. It is last as you are more likely to remember the first and last points and these are the two most important.

Carbohydrate in your diet is the real enemy, not fat. All the hysteria about saturated fat over the last few decades is probably just that, hysteria. This issue about carbohydrate particularly applies if you are overweight and have features of the metabolic syndrome with special attention to type two diabetes.

As you will now understand from earlier discussions, type two diabetes, where your body is resistant to the effects of insulin so that the insulin doesn't work properly, is present in epidemic and increasing proportions in our society. Remember type two diabetes is not a lack of insulin, like type one diabetes, it is a failure of the body to respond to the insulin, which is often already present in large amounts. Consequently your blood sugar rises and you need other medication, or extra insulin as injections, to control the blood sugar level keeping it down in the normal range. If you ate no carbohydrate at all it is likely you would not need to take anything for your diabetes. This is assuming we are discussing early type two diabetics. Late in type two diabetes the insulin levels sometimes do fall as the pancreas fails or if you like wears out. Under no circumstances do these comments apply to people with type one diabetes, this is a completely different disease. Remember don't stop or reduce the dose of your insulin if you have either type of diabetes without medical advice.

Generally speaking, the disease type two diabetes, and up to a point the whole metabolic syndrome, implies your body cannot handle simple carbohydrate which we also call sugar. In other words if your exercise level remains static this is best considered a "sugar overload" situation. This means any complex carbohydrate (long chain of sugar molecules) that is broken down into single sugar molecules (individual links of the chain) for you to absorb, you are going to have trouble with. Perhaps not as much trouble as with pure sugar where the links of the chain are already single, but trouble all the same. Remember the glycaemic index (GI) of a food just gives you a measure of how rapidly this sugar is absorbed into the blood, in other words how rapidly you can chop the chain up into individual links. Sure the lower the glycaemic index of a food is the better, as you don't want those sugar molecules hitting you like a cartridge of lead pellets fired out of a shotgun all at once, but it is still carbohydrate, the one thing your body cannot deal with in its current state. Brown rice is still rice, it is just more slowly absorbed and broken down than white rice. Wholemeal flour is still flour, it is just a slower acting poison than white flour.

Now diabetes specialists, dieticians and nutritionists have been telling diabetics for years that they must have carbohydrate in their diet and it just matters what type of carbohydrate they have, in other words low GI or complex carbohydrate is OK. They then give you tablets and injections like insulin to control the blood sugar and we wonder why diabetics never lose weight! I clearly remember being told many times as a trainee doctor that once you begin a type two diabetic on insulin they never lose weight. Well how can the poor sods lose weight when you have just given them something to force their bodies to make some more fat and to increase their appetite?! I would have to confess that, although this is not my specialty area, I think this strategy is very seriously flawed in logic and I think this alternate viewpoint is slowly gaining traction. If you have the condition of carbohydrate poisoning why on Earth would you take more carbohydrate?! Surely this is the same logic as treating a patient with alcoholic poisoning with more alcohol?! Sure many alcoholics do this but they end up dead. I have seen this happen more times than I can remember as this really is my area of specialist interest as a Gastroenterologist. Liver disease is part of my area of expertise. Fatty liver disease, or if you like the earliest stage of type two diabetes, is best considered carbohydrate poisoning of the liver. Looking at the liver under the microscope the fatty liver disease from carbohydrate poisoning is indistinguishable from early alcoholic poisoning of the liver, they look absolutely identical.

So, from my perspective, advising a type two diabetic to have complex carbohydrate instead of sugar is essentially the same thing as advising an alcoholic to drink wine instead of straight whisky. Sure it is not as bad but it is still poison to them and it will still do them harm. You are just ensuring they never "kick the habit." The only difference is that their "habit" is carbohydrate not alcohol. We thus ensure they will be diabetic till the day they die. With this advice we are just making sure this day will be sooner rather than later.

Now I am not saying that you can have no carbohydrate as a diabetic or even as an overweight individual. I am saying just that if you are having trouble losing weight, or controlling your diabetes, and going to cut anything out this should be what you cut out first. It is the real enemy and you should probably be eating a low carbohydrate diet rather than a low fat diet if you need to choose. The term "healthy low fat diet" is likely to be a myth where you are concerned.

So if you need that glucose, a form of sugar, to run your brain and keep you alive, where do you get it from when you are on a low carbohydrate diet?

Well several sources. Firstly it is very hard to exclude all carbohydrate from your diet so no matter how hard you try some is going to slip through. A low carbohydrate diet also, by definition, means you must be eating something else if you are eating at all. One component of those other things is protein. You can make glucose from protein, just not as efficiently as you can make it from complex carbohydrates such as potatoes or rice. Still you will get more than enough glucose, especially if you are diabetic. If you simply replace large amounts of carbohydrate in your diet with large amounts of protein you may still need some medication to cope with the glucose produced from the protein. This is why I want your doctor involved in any decisions related to medication changes.

So if it is that simple where is the evidence to prove this point? Well you may be surprised to learn there is so much of it out there I could bury you in the scientific and medical journal articles proving this point. Let us just look briefly at one study, published in 2003 where Doctors took 132 severely obese subjects, 39% of whom had type two diabetes. Now this study only went for six months which is a short time in your life but it makes the point well. Subjects were randomised to either a carbohydrate restricted or a fat restricted diet for the duration of the study. Those on the carbohydrate restricted diet lost more than three times as much weight as those on the fat restricted diet, an average of 5.8 kg compared with 1.9 kg. The low carbohydrate diet was better tolerated (likely easier to adhere to) than the low fat diet in that far more subjects in the low fat diet group dropped out of the study. Those on the low carbohydrate diet had a greater reduction in harmful blood fats (triglycerides) and more of an improvement in insulin sensitivity, the latter the best measure over all of their diabetes and the metabolic syndrome. So why do many Doctors and other health professionals still tell patients to follow a "healthy" low fat diet to achieve weight loss or diabetic control when we have proven long ago that this approach doesn't work?

Beats me!

---

*Fred Samaha et al, New England Journal of Medicine, May 22 2003*

Is a very low carb diet healthy long term? The answer is we don't know. So please don't be too extreme here in your dietary choices in the long term. What we do know is that a very high carbohydrate diet is certainly very unhealthy if you don't make use of it and you store it up for later. This is one of the most important messages in the book.

I would advise not to have a huge amount of protein to replace the carbs as this, at least in rat and mice models, is not a good thing long term, or if you like for the duration of their lives. The duration of your life is what I am discussing with you. So what is a safe amount of protein in your diet long term, I say again "we don't know." I would try to stay below 1.5-2g per Kg body weight per day, at least in the long term or until we know the answer.

Animal (saturated) fats have got a lot of bad press over the last 50 years which as I have said may not be fully, if at all warranted, but again I would like you focusing on the fats we think are healthier such as vegetable oils, for example nut and fish oils. This certainly does not mean no to animal fat just don't overdo this either. I would rather you had another piece of steak with your salad than a serve the potato salad or chips. If you have to pour a lot of olive oil, with the balsamic vinegar, over your salad to ensure you feel full and satisfied with the meal so be it. It works try it. Just don't have that piece of bread or a potato and NEVER use prepacked sweet (loaded with sugar) processed salad dressings.

There is one thing that I think is becoming harder and harder to ignore here. Carbohydrate, particularly simple carbohydrates (sugars), are likely to be the number one enemy to your achieving and maintaining weight loss. They are the number one enemy in your achieving control of your diabetes. Please keep reminding yourself of this and act accordingly! As you well know "Actions speak louder than words."

There is an excellent recent review of this topic in the medical literature but please be aware I am being selective here - quoting articles which agree with my personal view point. Having said this the article is well argued and an evidence based review of the medical literature. They make a number of salient points all backed up by the evidence available, which they reference in the article. They are referring primarily to the management of diabetes however I believe much of this view point can be extrapolated to the rest of the metabolic syndrome. These points include;

1.  Hyperglycaemia (high blood glucose) is the most salient feature of diabetes. Dietary carbohydrate restriction has the greatest effect on decreasing blood sugar levels.

2.  During the recent epidemics of obesity and type 2 diabetes (1974-2000, USA), calorific increases in this society have been almost entirely due to increased carbohydrate intake.

3.  The benefits of dietary carbohydrate restriction do not require weight loss. (for example reduction in blood sugar or blood fat levels)

4.  Although weight loss is not required for benefit, no dietary intervention has been shown to be more effective than carbohydrate restriction for weight loss.

5. Adherence to low-carbohydrate diets is at least as good as adherence to any other dietary interventions and is frequently significantly better. In other words you are more likely to tolerate and stick to this type of dietary change.

6. Replacement of carbohydrate with protein is generally beneficial in these diabetic patients. Protein replacement of carbohydrate is associated with more weight loss, more body fat loss and higher resting metabolic rate. This is when compared to low fat diets or diets replacing the carbohydrate with fat alone, which is the usual approach in "low carb" type diets.

7. Dietary total and saturated fat intake do not correlate with risk for cardiovascular disease.

8. Restricting dietary carbohydrate is more effective than restricting dietary fat in lowering the levels of saturated fats in the blood. (Remember the saturated fat level in the blood, not the diet, correlates with the risk of heart and vascular disease)

9. Lack of control of blood sugar level in type 2 diabetes is the best predictor of damage to large and small arteries in the body. Remember this "damage" can then manifest itself as strokes, heart attacks, kidney disease and other "complications" of diabetes.

10. Dietary carbohydrate restriction is the most effective method (other than starvation) for reducing serum triglycerides levels

(another form of harmful fat in the blood) and increasing high-density lipoprotein levels (good or protective type of cholesterol in the blood).

11. Patients with type 2 diabetes on carbohydrate restricted diets reduce and frequently eliminate the need for medication. Patients with type 1 diabetes usually require lower insulin doses. (Remember if you change your medication dosage please do it with your doctors input)

12. The side effects of intensive glucose lowering by dietary carbohydrate restriction, if any, are much less severe than the side effects of intensive drug treatment to control blood glucose in diabetes. You having any trouble with drug side effects such as diarrhoea or nausea from your metformin? Putting on weight with your insulin?

To date there are no long term studies in humans on the safety of adopting a long term very low carbohydrate approach to diabetes, that I am aware of. If one is coming to reassure you it is probably years away. The benefits of this diet on the other hand are well documented and immediate.

There are countless studies showing a high carbohydrate diet in the absence of adequate exercise, is very bad for you. At the time of publication, and based on current evidence, I advise my patients with features of the metabolic syndrome to follow a low carbohydrate diet.

To quote one of the authors of this recent evidence based review; "At the end of our clinic day, we go home thinking, "The clinical improvements are so large and so obvious, why don't other doctors understand? (The concept of) Carbohydrate restriction is easily grasped by patients."

You read the article and make up your own mind but I say again: Do not change your medication doses or go on a very low carbohydrate diet without discussing this with your doctor. Both your medication and a low carb diet are effective in reducing your blood glucose level and if you do them both together you are at significant risk of inducing episodes of hypoglycaemia (dangerously low blood glucose levels). Changes will need to be done carefully and your blood sugar monitored.

---

*Richard Feinman et al, Nutrition 31 (2015) 1-13*

# PRACTICAL EXAMPLES OF WHAT TO DO

MOST OF THESE points are relatively self-explanatory, however I would like to walk you through some simple examples to get you started and to organise your daily routine.

When we talk about processed foods, I am not trying to totally eradicate them from your diet, just to get you to open your eyes and actually read the labels, so don't forget your glasses when you go shopping! If you use common sense, some are clearly okay and this includes things like unsweetened dairy foods, fresh frozen vegetables, tinned fish in water (rather than oil and preferably without added salt), tinned tomatoes and many others. Your radar should be watching out for added sugar and fat or oil. You should also avoid salt if possible because of its negative effects on blood pressure, although it will not affect your weight.

Eating upside down is another important issue and if you can do this you are more likely to succeed. Let's start with breakfast. Now you can have a large standard breakfast with several courses and not feel guilty. Ideally, I would like you to have your "evening" type meal for breakfast and by this I mean your chicken, meat or fish curry and brown rice (or preferably chopped vegetables-especially if we are going low carb). This is most likely too big a jump for most of you. So if you want to stick with your muesli (preferably homemade and not sweetened or fried/baked, with your oats, dry roasted pumpkin seeds, chopped unsalted nuts, sunflower seeds, small amount of chopped dried fruits, shredded coconut etc.) with milk then that's Okay. True, it is easier to buy this, but be careful to read what is in it and how it is prepared. You can follow this with a couple of slices of toast with scrambled eggs on them as well if you like, preferably without butter. Now that's about 160 calories for the cup of muesli, 80 for the cup of milk, 250 for the scrambled eggs, taking into account the use of some oil and cheese and fried mushrooms and tomatoes as well, 160 for the 2 slices of bread, giving you about 700-800 calories for breakfast, including your 2 cups of coffee without sugar. Sorry, forgot to tell you—you've given up sugar. Milk's okay but only a splash. Also remember any "frying" is a non-stick pan with a quick spray of oil. Now if you have diabetes or this just does not seem to be working for you with respect to weight loss, then I am afraid we will have to lose the carbs here. By this I mean the muesli and the toast. This can be replaced by a larger cooked breakfast including alternatives such as ham, meat, fish or another protein source as well as the eggs and   low carb vegetables. For example a zucchini split down the middle and cooked in the pan with the mushrooms. If you are having the fish curry for breakfast then there is definitely no rice, just the grated steamed cauliflower to put it on.

Now at morning break, you are hopefully not hungry after your large breakfast so go for a walk if you must to avoid food at work. If you simply cannot, then have a hot chocolate with of two teaspoons of cocoa, one of inulin fibre supplement and a splash of milk. The cocoa will supress your appetite within about one hour and the inulin fibre in about 6 hours, helping reduce your food intake later in the day.

Lunch is a salad sandwich which includes a slice of cheese or meat/fish, this is about 350 calories, with your hot chocolate, tea or coffee. If you are diabetic there is no bread, just a larger salad with your meat, fish or cheese. Oil and vinegar are fine in the dressing.

By the afternoon break, if you get one, hopefully the inulin and cocoa will have done their job but it is reasonable to have another cup. Cocoa is actually very good for you for many reasons as discussed earlier but I would not take large amounts in the evening because of the caffeine-like effect of the theobromine that the cocoa contains.

Now the evening meal is likely to be where problems will arise. If the cocoa and the inulin fibre leave you relatively full, then try to avoid this meal altogether. That is the best option. Though this can be difficult for social and other reasons as discussed. If you want a hot meal then try one serve (100g) of fish, chicken or low fat beef/pork, this is between 150-200 calories. You don't know what 100g is? Well what do you think you brought those new kitchen scales for? If you are baking this in the oven with a light spray of rice bran or other oil, then there are numerous vegetables you can add. Remember, these days you do not pour oil in a pan, you spray it, and it is okay to spray a bit on the non-stick baking pan and on top of the vegetables, to brown them. Use one of the pump up pressure devices you refill yourself, not spray cans. We have enough landfill already.

The following examples are for one cup of chopped vegetables. Broccoli, cauliflower, capsicum and asparagus are about 30 calories per cup, green leafy vegetables like spinach and lettuce are less than 10 calories, celery is about 15 calories per cup, squash, zucchini and mushrooms are about 20 calories per cup. Onions are a bit higher at 50 calories per cup and sweeter vegetables like carrots 60 calories per cup and should not be considered if you are diabetic. By the way, you don't eat pumpkin or potatoes, sweet or otherwise, any more, you have kicked the habit. Remember however, onions are full of inulin which may inhibit your appetite and capsicum may increase your metabolic rate, offsetting the higher energy value. So if you steam a few cups of vegetables or you bake/fry them with the fish/chicken/meat you will end up with about a 300 calorie evening meal. Add as much garlic and chilli or other flavour enhancers as you like. Don't forget to add the 80 calories in your one glass of wine. If you wait about an hour, the protein in the meal will make you feel satisfied. What do you do for the hour you feel hungry after the small evening meal? You go for a walk, even if it has to be on a machine while you watch the TV or listen to music.

This totals about 1500 calories for the whole day which with a minor few slip ups goes to 1600-1800 and WILL make you lose weight, especially if you leave out the carbs. How did I work out all the calorie counts? Simple, I used google and it took me about 2 minutes. Just google "calories in one serve of x." Now you can write it down in your calorie counting record for the day, along with your weight this week.

Now let's just look at a slip up that really matters. Got home exhausted and stressed, you were a bit hungry and found a 200g chocolate bar in the pantry. Oops, ate the whole thing! That was 1100 calories, nearly your total daily allowance in one bar of chocolate! Stuffs the whole day up doesn't it. Don't have it in the pantry and don't buy it at the shops! I say again, you don't plan to fail so don't fail to plan!

Now for exercise, you have a few choices. If you are going to have a big breakfast then you probably need to get up an hour earlier in the mornings and go for a brisk walk/jog/bike ride with your neighbour/friend for 45 minutes each morning to work up your appetite. Alternatively, you could do some weight lifting exercises at the gym or with the weights and the stretch straps you got for yourself to use at home. It is better to do this sort of exercise on an empty stomach before breakfast to avoid heartburn and reflux. Making breakfast may take you a bit longer but if it is a chicken curry with chopped vegetables you could have pre-packaged and frozen it already. Just needs the microwave while you have a shower after your walk.

Remember the couch you used to sit on in the evening was replaced with the exercise bike or running machine so when you watch the news or other things on the TV in the evening you get another 30-60 minutes of walking, jogging or riding instead of eating dessert. You had a small main so exercise is OK. If it safe to do so, you could go for another walk outside as an alternative but take that poor dog of yours, it needs the exercise too.

Aiming for seven hours of sleep is easy enough but may require going to bed earlier as you are now getting up earlier. Only one glass of wine or beer to quench your thirst with the hot curried food you are now eating on your smaller plates. Reducing alcohol in the evening is very important for good quality sleep and obviously reduces calories. If you can add a 5/2 type diet plan with 2 days of markedly restricted calorie intake you are sure to succeed. The other points are self-explanatory.

If you feel very guilty because you have just eaten the chocolate bar, and have nothing important to do for the next 8 hours, take 2-3 teaspoons of magnesium sulphate (Epsom salts, bath salts) in 2-3 glasses of water. This can do as the rest of your evening meal. Don't plan to leave the house. The laxative effect will help to minimise how much you absorb of the calories, and you will think twice before you eat that chocolate again! Nothing like a bit of self-flagellation! You may even start to associate, subconsciously, eating chocolate with bad diarrhoea and it will stop you even wanting to eat chocolate again. The brain is "plastic" and can be manipulated and retrained. Try it. It works.

# SUMMARY

I F YOU FOLLOW these guidelines you will lose weight. I don't want you to "try" to do some of the 17, I want you to "do" all of them. Remember you must choose between being a player or a spectator here. There may be some easier options coming but they are not here yet, so in the interim prove to those weight loss surgeons you do not need them. You can do it yourself! Tell the surgeons they can take an early retirement! Draw yourself up a chart so you can tick all the boxes. Place the chart on the wall or refrigerator door where it is very conspicuous. It must be in plain sight. The details in this book, such as the chemicals which control appetite, where they come from and how they work, are unimportant. They are just mentioned for those who are interested. What is important is that you understand the general principles.

You are likely to live longer as a result of your efforts and if, like me, you are not sure you are going to a better place, then I would recommend hanging around here as long as possible. You will also live a much healthier, more active life and as a result hope-fully be able to get up to much more mischief. This is about the quality of your life, not just the quantity.

You will benefit greatly from having a good local doctor who will support you in your endeavour, in conjunction with the book. I would strongly suggest you ask your doctor if you can work out a program and see them at least monthly for the first year. You must stick to the program. They can mobilise other troops such as dieticians if you need help understanding the issues relating to food types and calorie counting or psychologists who may be able to help with motivation. This will give you the opportunity to ask them any questions you may have on the important principles in the book, to document your weight loss, to encourage and congratulate you, and reassess things like your blood pressure and your diabetes if applicable. Hopefully you will be able to come off many of your tablets in the longer term. The visits will give you the opportunity to prove to your doctor what both of you had always felt was impossible. That you could do it! It will be a good feeling.

As I have described, there are many options you have available for tackling weight loss. These include what you eat, when you eat, why you eat, how quickly you eat and many other things. I would hope you use all the information in this book to your advantage to give you the best possible chance of success. Please remember that what you put in your mouth is the most important issue by far. If you remember nothing else, I want you to change the way you think about this. Humour me for a short while longer and imagine the world has come to an end. There is no more food. What you have to live on is what you have stored in your pantry. When you run out of food you die. I am sure in this situation you will try and get the food to last as long as possible to maximise the time you have left alive, hoping something or someone comes along to save you.

What most of you don't seem to realise is that your life in reality is actually very similar to this. There really is a finite amount you are able to eat in your life before you die. If you eat it all by the age of 45 you will end up very obese and you are likely to have a heart attack or develop bowel cancer. You are likely to die young. If you eat this finite amount of food slowly and in moderation you will not be obese and you are much less likely to develop the Western diseases that we call the metabolic syndrome. Diseases that cause so many premature deaths. Consequently, you are more likely to live until you are 85-90 years of age, getting a lot more quantity and quality of life. All for the same amount of food.

The obvious extrapolation of this argument is that every mouthful you take, takes you one step closer to your grave. I'm afraid, speaking generally, this is true, much as you might like to deny it. Remember this every time you eat. It goes both ways. If you starve animals such as rats they live 30% longer than normally fed non-obese rats. If you overfeed them you can shorten their lives by 50% compared with normally fed non-obese rats.

There is no question you will get to your grave, we all will, nothing is more certain. Your choice here is how quickly you want to get there. Exercise is best thought of as the one way you have of taking the excess food credits you have eaten back out of you and putting them back in the stock pile for use at a later date. This may buy you more time.

If you don't like this analogy, then try the next one.

Your life is a bit like jumping off a skyscraper. There is no question you are going to hit the pavement, just as there is no question that one day you are going to die. The problem is while you are falling, or passing through life in this example, you feel completely relaxed and weightless, you have no realisation there are any problems at all. If anyone sticks their head out of a window of the skyscraper as you sail past and says, "How's life?" you will reply, "Great thanks, all is going really well!" The problem is once you have hit the pavement there is no turning back. You cannot step back out of your grave. This book is your parachute. You do have a problem. You do need to use your parachute. Wake up and open your eyes: this is not a dream, it is reality!

Remember, this quest does not end in a month or a year, it is a lifestyle change. It is for good.

I would wish you luck but I hope by now you realise your success or failure in this quest has nothing whatsoever to do with luck. It has nothing whatsoever to do with magic. It has nothing whatsoever to do with other people. It has everything to do with you! The ball is in your court.

A friend of mine who is a weight loss surgeon, has spoken to me about this book several times. He wishes me all the best but feels strongly I am wasting my time with this quest. It is his view that 98% of you out there will fail to lose weight in the long term without surgery, and to be fair there is literature to support his view. He, and I suspect his colleagues, have near to zero faith in you achieving your goal without surgery, or 2% of you at best.

If we all shared this view then clearly there is no point in your attempting weight loss. There is no point in your having read this book. The game is lost before it has even begun.

Well, I for one do not share this view and I trust you don't either. I cannot prove him, or his colleagues in the area of weight loss surgery wrong. To be fair they do a great job when all else fails. It is just that, where YOU are concerned, we are not going to fail. You are going to succeed and prove this commonly held view is incorrect. It would be great if we could reverse the figures so only 2% of people needed to fall back on the surgeons, not 98%, wouldn't it?! I can only help those of you who want to be helped, which unfortunately is not everyone in need.

For those of you who do want help:

It IS possible. I know you can do it!

I do have faith in you!

# ABOUT THE AUTHOR:

STEPHEN FAIRLEY IS a Medical Specialist in Gastroenterology and Liver disease with a particular interest in the management of obesity. He holds a Bachelor of Medicine and Surgery from the University of Melbourne, is a Fellow of the Royal Australian College of Physicians and is a member of the American Gastroenterological Association and the Gastroenterological Society of Australia. He currently works, in private and public practice, and as a Clinical Senior lecturer with The James Cook University Medical School, Townsville Australia.

He has more than twenty years of experience in specialist medical practice and teaching in Townsville where he lives with his wife, Carol, and their four children.

## Cover Illustration:

Harry McGlone

www.ingramcontent.com/pod-product-compliance
Lightning Source LLC
Chambersburg PA
CBHW060535210326
41519CB00014B/3225